". . . a formidable yet worthwhile and pioneering task in a difficult, unpopular area of disturbed human behavior . . . Interesting, readable, original . . . Of value to begin to understand these age-old complex sexual behaviors."

—Domeena C. Renshaw, M.D.
Journal of American Medical Association

"This is an affliction that affects large numbers of men and women."

—Phil Donahue

"Patrick Carnes has pioneered a treatment for sex addiction."

—*USA Today*

"What's significant about the [sexual addiction] concept is that it gives people a label for understanding their very puzzling and destructive patterns of sexual behavior."

—John Grace, therapist
St. Paul Pioneer Press/Dispatch

"Patrick Carnes is the acknowledged expert in a field that until recently didn't exist."

—*Philadelphia*

"I just want to say thank you for understanding me. It's the first time that I felt my problem crystallized for me. I not only [speak] as a professional, but as an addict. It's the first step for me."

—Anonymous

Other books by Patrick Carnes, Ph.D. . . .

The Betrayal Bond: Breaking Free of Exploitive Relationships (Health Communications, 1997)

Contrary to Love: Helping the Sexual Addict (Hazelden, 1989)

Don't Call It Love: Recovery from Sexual Addiction (Bantam, 1992)

Facing the Shadow: Starting Sexual and Relationship Recovery (Gentle Path Press, 2001)

A Gentle Path through the Twelve Steps: The Classic Guide for All People in the Process of Recovery (Hazelden, 1993)

Open Hearts: Renewing Relationships with Recovery, Romance, and Reality, with Mark R. Laaser and Debra J. Laaser (Gentle Path Press, 1999)

In the Shadows of the Net: Breaking Free of Compulsive Online Sexual Behavior, with Elizabeth Griffin, David L. Delmonico, and Joseph M. Moriarity (Hazelden, 2001)

Sexual Anorexia: Overcoming Sexual Self-Hatred, with Joseph M. Moriarity (Hazelden, 1997)

Out of the Shadows

Understanding Sexual Addiction

Patrick Carnes, Ph.D.

Third Edition

Hazelden Publishing
Center City, Minnesota 55012-0176
hazelden.org/bookstore

Library of Congress Cataloging-in-Publication Data
Carnes, Patrick, 1944-
    Out of the shadows : understanding sexual addiction/Patrick
    Carnes.--3rd ed.
       p. cm.
    First ed. originally published in 1983 by CompCare under the title:
    The sexual addiction.
    ISBN 978-1-56838-621-8 (paperback)
       1. Sex addiction. I. Carnes, Patrick, 1944- . Sexual addiction. II. Title.

RC560.S43 C38 2001
616.85'83--dc21   2001024399

Editor's note
All the stories in this book are based on actual experiences. The names and details have been changed to protect the privacy of the people involved. In some cases, composites have been created.

This book is intended as a guide to understanding both the sexual addiction and the Twelve Steps as a means of recovery. Neither the book, its author, nor its publisher endorses any specific Twelve Step group for sexual compulsiveness. Readers are encouraged to investigate thoroughly any such group as to its appropriateness for them.

The Twelve Steps are reprinted and adapted with permission of Alcoholics Anonymous World Services, Inc. (AAWS). Permission to reprint and adapt the Twelve Steps does not mean that AAWS has reviewed or approved the contents of this publication, or that AAWS necessarily agrees with the views expressed herein. AA is a program of recovery from alcoholism *only*—use of the Twelve Steps in connection with programs and activities which are patterned after AA, but which address other problems, does not imply otherwise.

19 18 17 16 15   13 14 15 16 17

Cover design by Theresa Gedig
Interior design by Stanton Publication Services, Inc.
Typesetting by Tursso Companies

This book is written to help the many addicts who have been afraid to admit their pain. One of the strongest bonds of the addiction is its secrecy. Perhaps, with the secret broken, addicts can know the peace and self-acceptance that comes with knowing *it can be talked about.*

Contents

Illustrations

Figures

Preface to the 2001 Edition

I had given my friend Sherod Miller an early draft of what was eventually to become the first edition of *Out of the Shadows*. Sherod, whose organization had published an earlier book of mine, was a respected author, with his *Couples Communication* in seventeen foreign editions. I really wanted his opinion of the manuscript. During dinner in a Minneapolis hotel, Sherod and I discussed my writing. As we talked, it became clear that the editorial state of the book was not his concern.

He finally looked at me and said, "Pat, this book is going to change your life."

A shudder of premonition went through me—something that always seems to happen when an inescapable reality in my life is reached. I remember quietly dismissing the significance of Sherod's statement by assuring him that I was prepared to face whatever happened. Twenty years later to the month, I can say that nothing, not Sherod's comment or anything else, could have prepared me for what happened. And, yes, the book did transform my life.

The book actually appeared in December 1983, entitled *The Sexual Addiction*. I have never agonized as much over any task before or since. I joked that I really did not know how the book was written. What I meant was that this book came from some quiet place of certitude within me—and, in that sense, it was not about me or any abilities that I might possess. It was more about a truth that would not rest until expressed. I simply gave voice to the perception of sexual pain I saw in struggling people.

Shortly after the book was published, it became clear that the book needed to be retitled. So much shame existed about the illness that readers found it difficult even to purchase the book with the title *The Sexual Addiction*. Renamed *Out of the*

Shadows, with *Understanding Sexual Addiction* as a subtitle, the book began to sell. And with the broader audience, those changes my friend Sherod talked about began to happen.

First came the mail. The book had tapped into a deep undercurrent of sexual trauma in our culture. People needed to talk about their pain. So they wrote letters. Most wrote because they were grateful. Many were struggling with inadequate resources. There were people in prisons with no help, people who had little Twelve Step support in their communities, and others who needed help and could not find treatment or therapists.

All walks of life were represented in these letters, as well as all kinds of sexual addiction problems. There was the woman whose husband failed to return after he had gone to his office on a Sunday in order "to catch up." She and her eight-year-old daughter found him in a rest room, dead of autoerotic asphyxiation. She wrote that she understood the addiction and how he got there. But her greatest problem now was how to deal with her daughter—the image of her father hanging by his belt in the midst of piles of pornography continued to haunt her.

Another came from the daughter of a sex addict who had died of a heart attack. Her mother and sisters were stunned to find that he was simultaneously married to two other women who also had children. Her agony was about her rage damming up her grief.

A Native American man wrote about how sex addiction can parallel alcoholism on the reservations. As a therapist, an alcoholic, and a recovering sex addict, he wrote with the authority of someone who had been there. He described how young Indian children had been taken out of abusive families and placed in boarding schools. There they were sexually abused by the older children, and the older ones were, in turn, being abused by the staff. As he wrote, "It was no accident I ended up where I did." His efforts to advocate for kids were, at best, met by apathy and more often by outrage on the part of government agencies and even the tribal council. The good news is that his individual voice—unwelcome as it was—made a difference.

I heard from a professional who told this painful story. In the early 1980s, his exhibitionism was so bad that he knew it was only a matter of time before his arrest. He so feared how this would affect his wife and children that he plotted his suicide. He had tried all the therapies available and felt there were no alternatives for him. So he took out large insurance policies and planned a car "accident." Filled with pain and feeling suicidal, he spotted a copy of *Out of the Shadows*. It offered enough hope for him to seek a Twelve Step group and therapy. Seven years later, he has over six years of problem-free behavior, a successful career, and a supportive family. He thinks about the old days in the street only about twice a year. And when he does, whatever power the compulsion still has is overwhelmed by gratitude.

Then there were the letters from the elderly. One woman told me that her husband, who himself was a therapist, discovered the book a few months before he died. She said it was "like gold" to him. Knowing about the addiction brought him peace. Similarly, another woman wrote about how her husband had been disabled by a car accident when he was fifty-four, just as she was about to leave him because of his womanizing. Because he was an invalid, she instead chose to stay with him. Upon his death twenty years later, she was amazed to find two decades of letters written since the accident to women she did not know about. Finding *Out of the Shadows* helped her separate her grief over the loss of a loved one from that other grief that comes with feeling betrayed.

Out of the Shadows started a conversation about the dark side of our sexuality. In the early struggle to educate people about alcoholism, we had to deal mostly with extreme prejudice, ignorance, and pain. The subject of sex addiction, however, tapped into some of our most primitive terrors. The reactions to it, therefore, are exponential. Unlike alcohol, sex is at the core of our identities. To understand our sexuality in new ways forces a shift in our self-perceptions.

All suffering contains gifts. And sex addiction is no different. It has expanded dramatically our knowledge of addictions in general. As a result of our increasing awareness of sex addiction, we know more about the addictive family system, the neurochemistry of addictions, the role of child abuse in addictions, and the impact of shame on addictive behavior. As eating disorders have helped us understand healthy eating, so sex addiction has provided us with new perspectives on healthy sex. The women's movement, the men's movement, pornography, AIDS, sex offenders, sexual harassment—many of our most divisive or controversial issues are sexual ones, and they take on new shades of meaning within the context of sex addiction.

Sex addiction itself has not been without controversy. But the debate has shifted from concerns about whether or not such an illness exists to how, and in what forms, and for what reasons.

Sex addicts have taught me much since *Out of the Shadows* was written. My book *Don't Call It Love* (Bantam, 1992) describes the course of recovery for more than a thousand sex addicts and their partners. These books are very different. The science of the second simply validates the spirit of the first. In this third edition I have woven some of the most important findings into the original text.

Since the original *Out of the Shadows* was published, the

sexual landscape has changed dramatically. First, there was
the AIDS epidemic, which sharply underlined how sex could
be compulsive. To have unprotected sex with someone you
know has AIDS is a self-destructive act. And yet that story
was all too common. Our culture learned that it was not a
"gay" problem or even a "male" problem, but a disease
whose impact has devastated whole cultures. And it high-
lighted the problem of sex addiction. *Sexual Addiction and
Compulsivity: The Journal of Treatment and Prevention* has
recently devoted an entire issue to AIDS and sex addiction as
a worldwide problem.

Then there was former President Clinton and the intern
Monica Lewinsky. Out of all the pain involved in that era
some remarkable events occurred. Suddenly decades of
research became available through journalists who were
using words like "compartmentalization," "anxiety reduction," and "loss of control." In their effort to understand presidential behavior, they took what clinicians and researchers
had learned about sex addiction and pumped it into the
national discussion. The controversy generated a gigantic
leap in awareness. If we were thirty to forty years behind the
public understanding of alcoholism, we suddenly were only
ten to fifteen years behind now.[1]

Almost simultaneously came the cybersex revolution.
Sexual activity on the Internet has fundamentally altered our
sexuality—and most professionals are unsure as to how or
even how much. Barriers and obstacles to sexual exploration
were literally obliterated overnight. The sex industry developed technology core to the Internet for distribution of
pornography. Its investment is now the third largest economic sector on the Internet. Considering that there are cur-
rently more than one hundred thousand pornography Web
sites and more than two hundred new ones introduced daily,

surfing the Internet for pornography has become a problem
for many. Most pornography is downloaded between 9:00
A.M. and 5:00 P.M., making it a corporate problem.

This does not account for all the other sexual activities on
the Internet, including chat rooms, news groups, escort services, and special interest sites. As one Stanford researcher
working with MSNBC data observed, there are now people
struggling with sexual compulsivity who never would have
been if not for the Internet.[2] About 40 percent of these sex
addicts are women. A case can be made that this has opened
up our culture to new attitudes and sexual understanding.
Clearly for some, it has been more than they bargained for.

Most sex addicts today struggle with some kind of activity
on the Internet. Since it has now become the great facilitator
of sexual acting out, this updated third edition of *Out of the
Shadows* includes an entire chapter on cybersex addiction.
Readers who wish to learn more about this particular aspect
of sexual compulsion are urged to read *In the Shadows of the
Net: Breaking Free of Compulsive Online Sexual Behavior*, which
was written with the help of David Delmonico, Elizabeth
Griffin, and Joe Moriarity. I predict that cybersex will change
the rules for everything sexual. In truth, it probably already
has.

Today, to help sex addicts and sexual trauma patients therapists are using technology that we never dreamed possible
decades ago. Professional colleagues in hospitals and outpatient settings all over the world are doing creative and inno-
vative therapy. Forums now exist for clinicians and scientists to
share their findings. *Sexual Addiction and Compulsivity: The
Journal of Treatment and Prevention* has established itself as a
peer-reviewed medical journal. The National Council on Sexual
Addiction and Compulsivity (NCSAC), both nationally and in
its local state chapters, works diligently to help understand

this illness. NCSAC pulls together concerned citizens, professionals, and public leaders to reduce the stigma of addiction and educate the public. This book now contains an updated guide highlighting many important resources concerning sex addiction.

Through the years, therapists have come to understand what treatment works and what doesn't for sex addiction. Certain activities or "tasks," if they are carried out, make a huge difference in recovery. A companion workbook for beginning sexual recovery, *Facing the Shadow: Starting Sexual and Relationship Recovery* (Gentle Path Press, 2001), was in fact created to help focus on those activities that are beyond the scope of *Out of the Shadows*. The workbook would never have been possible without the original book, however.

That is, in fact, the problem I have had revising *Out of the Shadows*. My goal was to substantially update and revise the book so new readers will have what they need. Yet I wanted to preserve much of the original writing, which has proven so helpful. Frankly, I have wondered if I could improve upon it. I have, in fact, kept the original preface intact so the reader could see the point at which I started. In addition, I have elected to keep the original acknowledgments section, since these were the people who were around me then and supported me thoroughly in writing the original manuscript. So many others have helped me since then that it goes far beyond my abilities to summarize. So I let the starting point stand.

A story that puts all this in perspective is about two men who started a Twelve Step group in a southern state. After confiding to each other about their problem, one decided to go to treatment, and the other put the word out that they were beginning a Twelve Step meeting. For six Sunday evenings, the latter went alone to the church meeting room, set up the chairs, waited, and prayed. No one came. When the man returned from treatment and came to the meeting, a third member showed up. Now that meeting has grown so large that it has split many times and has developed wonderful traditions as a Twelve Step community. It all grew out of the faith of one and the action of the other. And so it has happened all over the country.

Yet the significance of this increasing understanding of sex addiction is more than the impact of individual stories, dramatic and encouraging as they are. There are those who make a case that the conflict, competition, and exploitation that erode our planet will not change until we, as humans, move into more collaborative and cooperative modes. Such a change in ecology starts with the most fundamental aspect of our relationships: our sexuality. We cannot evolve further until men and women treat each other differently. Respect for sexual preference, the protection of children from inappropriate and abusive behavior, the reduction of sexual shame, and the celebration of sexual joy will emerge naturally with a shift to nonpatriarchal, noncompetitive, and nonexploitive values about sex.

Each sex addict's recovery, therefore, is a clear contribution to the well-being of the planet. Sex addicts know how that recovery begins. For every addict a moment comes . . .

Preface to the 1983 Edition

This book represents an extraordinary pilgrimage for me. It started as an extended paper I wrote early in 1976 entitled "The Sex Offender: His Addiction, His Family, His Beliefs." Based on two years of experience of conducting outpatient groups with sex offenders, the paper developed the essential concepts that underlie this book and its companion volume, *Contrary to Love, Understanding Sexual Addiction, Part 2: Helping the Sexual Addict*.

The manuscript received wide circulation, but was never published. The paper served as a basis for many workshops and training events. Whole programs evolved based on its theoretical assumptions. Yet I remained reluctant to make the document a formal statement through publication. One reason for the reluctance was the realization that the sexual addiction extended to many men and women who had not done anything punishable by law. They were not "sex offenders," but suffered the same pathology. Also, in those early years there was insufficient documentation to support the concept of sexual compulsiveness as an addiction. Nor were there networks of programs available to help people who recognized their need. Most of all, I was afraid of the public reaction, which is always unpredictable in sexual matters. In short, it was an idea whose time had not come.

In 1976, a suburban hospital asked me to start an experimental program for chemically dependent families. Called the Family Renewal Center, the program required that all members of the family above age six participate in the 330-hour program. The theoretical constructs of the program originated in general systems theory, especially as it applied to families and the Twelve Steps of Alcoholics Anonymous. Within a short time, the entire staff realized that having all the family members present in the therapeutic process radically altered one's understanding of alcoholism and chemical dependency.

One of the many factors that stood out from a family perspective was that the addictive compulsivity had many forms other than alcohol and drug abuse. Also, the different forms—overeating, gambling, sexuality, buying, shoplifting—all shared a similar process. And in addition, within the family, addictions would be like overlays whose reinforcing shadows simply deepened the patterns of family pathology.

To further complicate matters, the reactions of family members to the multiaddiction patterns were as unhealthy as the coping of the addicts themselves. In understanding the family illness, we learned that each member must use a discipline such as the Twelve Steps as an ongoing antidote to the addictive process. Members of groups like Overeaters Anonymous and Gamblers Anonymous had already pioneered in applying the Twelve Steps to other addictions. Now the Family Renewal Center has extended its programming, based on the Twelve Steps, to sexual addiction, physical abuse, and food issues. The center also offers a series of wellness programs for families and couples.

Other than its offerings in chemical dependency, the center's sexual addiction programs are the most developed series of programs at the center. Sexual compulsivity was the first of the "other" addictions we tackled, by virtue of continuing my outpatient group work with offenders. Program development was intensified with a three-year grant from the National Center on Child Abuse and Neglect. Now the center offers family-oriented sexual abuse programs in both urban and rural sites, and similar programs are being set up in other regions of the country. The research efforts of that staff are, to my knowledge, the first extended and systematic articulation of the relationship between sexual compulsivity and chemical dependency that has a sound empirical base. Data and experience now exist that add credibility to the conceptualization done so many years ago.

Also, the growth of Twelve Step programs for sexual addiction across the country is a most encouraging development. The emerging network of groups not only provides help to people in pain, it also represents a milestone of public support, without which sexual addicts will never ultimately be able to escape their shame.

Over the years, the many discussions I have had with my colleagues and friends have made it difficult to isolate the genesis of concepts. I am indebted to them all for their contributions. Especially, I wish to thank

Miriam Ingebritson, whose creativity and critiques have often expanded my own limited paradigms.

Glenice Anderson, Dave Walsh, Tom Burton, Craig Nakken, Jim Michel, Shirley Carlson, Mary McBride, and the staff of the Family Renewal Center, whose advice, integrity, and support have been invaluable.

Allen Nohre, executive director of Fairview Treatment Centers, for his continuing support of my work.

Bill Mease, Warren Shaffer, Mark Davison, Richard Seely, Scott Moline, and Elaine Pfalzgraf, who as legal, police, or psychological professionals made important resources available.

Ann Golla and Janis Kromminga, who spent many long evening and weekend hours typing the manuscripts.

The members of Sexual Addicts Anonymous (SAA) whose reading and suggestions were the real test.

Professor Richard Clendenen and the alumni of the Juvenile Officers Institute of the University of Minnesota—if they had not confronted me, I would never have finished this book.

Diane DuCharme, whose early encouragement was indispensable.

Bonnie Hesse, who as editor could not have been more affirming.

Terri O'Grady, whose patient editing and care helped support the writing.

My children, David, Stefanie, Jennifer, and Erin, who have explained to me that this is one book they will not bring to school.

The people whose stories are reflected in these pages and who are the true pioneers.

With all of these people, my pilgrimage has not been alone, and for that I am truly grateful. With their help, what was begun in 1976 is now finished.

INTRODUCTION

A Moment Comes for Every Addict

▣   ▣   ▣

A moment comes for every addict when the consequences are so great or the pain is so bad that the addict admits life is out of control because of his or her sexual behavior. Some are news-making moments, such as the public censure when a congressman, minister, or professional figure is cited for unacceptable sexual behavior. Millions read the steamy news accounts and, despite their own prurience, make severe judgments about people who are sexual with children, who visit prostitutes, who commit homosexual acts in public toilets, or even who have affairs. A smaller audience—but much larger than most imagine—read each line fearing that the same public exposure could happen to them and judging themselves with the same unforgiving standards the public uses.

Some are dramatic moments:

- when the squad car pulls into the driveway and you know why they've come
- when you break off yet another relationship you never wanted to be in
- when your spouse succeeds in being elected to public office and is forced to resign because a sheriff sting caught you soliciting a minor over the Internet

- when your spouse announces the end of your marriage because of the latest discovery
- when your young son goes through your history files on your computer and sees all your pornography
- when your daughter's friend sees your photo in the mug shots at the police station and no one in your family knew
- when you have to leave your job because of a sexual entanglement with a person you never really liked anyway
- when your husband discovers e-mails to your lovers, who were his best friends and golfing companions
- when you are the first woman mayor of your city and one of your affairs is with the city manager, who happens to be the best friend of your husband, who will batter you if he finds out
- when the school counselor calls to inform you that your daughter does not want to come home because, after eight years, she no longer wants to be sexual, and you are being reported to child protection
- when you are a person with AIDS and you have unprotected anal sex with others every time you use cocaine and yet you continue to use
- when you have a car accident while exposing yourself

Some are secret moments known only to yourself:

- when you have to tell yet another lie that you almost believe yourself
- when the money you have spent on the last prostitute equals the amount for the new shoes your child needs
- when you see a person on the street you had been anonymously sexual with in a rest room
- when you make business travel decisions not on the

basis of company interests, but rather to accommodate
the affair that you are having

- when you tell someone "I love you," knowing full well
there are two others who also think they are the only
ones you love
- when you sit in a room full of people, three of whom
you have had sex with recently, and part of you fears
what they would do if they knew about the others, and
part of you gloats over your accomplishment
- when you say "I love you" because you know you are
going to go to bed with someone, yet you really don't
love or want to go to bed with that person
- when you cringe inside because your friends are laugh-
ing at a flasher joke, and you are one
- when you are an alcoholic completing treatment and
you realize that your time in the hospital was not only a
period free from chemicals, but also a time when you
were sexually at ease as well, and you never felt better
—yet you know that abstinence from alcohol will be
easy compared with stopping your sexual addiction

For most people these moments are followed by resolves
"never to do it again." Even as the promises are made, they
are rendered hollow by the echoes of the previous vows and
resolutions. Many are the addicts who have deeply wished
not to be sexual at all, thinking that state to be the only cure
for their compulsive feelings, thinking that by giving up their
sexuality they would be able to work, to love, and to enjoy
themselves like other people. Sexual addiction has been described as "the athlete's foot of the mind." It never goes away.
It is always asking to be scratched, promising relief. To
scratch, however, is to cause pain and to intensify the itch.

The "itch" is created in part by the rationalizations, lies, and beliefs about themselves carried deep within the sexual addicts. The husband, for example, who visits a prostitute and on his way home feels warm toward his wife and family tells himself that his time in the sauna really helps him to be more sensitive and loving to his family. At one level he knows the fallacy of his thinking, but chooses to ignore it in light of the immediate warm feelings. In contrast with the unfeeling exchanges of massage parlor life, the family does look much better. The cost to the family remains overlooked, however. So it is with the many beliefs, rationalizations, and myths that support addiction:

- I am oversexed.
- No one else is like me.
- I really did care for her/him.
- Just one more time won't hurt.
- I deserve it.
- It isn't so bad since everyone does it.
- She/he wanted, deserved, asked for it.

One of the greatest myths that allows the addict to repeat sexual behaviors is that it does not adversely affect other relationships, especially a marriage. In fact, one of the most common rationales for a married addict is "I do it in order to stay in the marriage." In reality, though, the marriage is often characterized by diminishing intimacy, sensitivity, and sexuality. The corollary myth is that the family does not know about the secret sexual life. Yet, at one level, family members always do know—even the children.

The facts are that, like all other addictions, the sexual addiction is rooted in a complex web of family and marital relationships. This interdependent web is truly a system in which a number of things act together to form one function, like a biological system or even a computer system. The system is governed by definite rules that, in the addict's case, confirm much of what he or she holds to be true in the crazy myths and beliefs which support the addiction. Also, all member parts have a functional relationship; that is, each person affects every other person. Nothing happens in isolation in this or any other system.

For the addict, part of therapy is to discover the role of the previous generation in the addiction. The exhibitionist who learns that his father, two uncles, and two cousins were also exhibitionists becomes keenly aware of how the "sins" of one generation are visited upon the next. Yet for years he was convinced he was the only one afflicted with the compulsion—a myth that added to the shame and pain at the core of his addiction. Many addicts find that the patterns of compulsion are learned quite early in the form of abuse, seduction, or simply witnessing compulsiveness in others.

Family members also have their parts in the system. The spouse who has learned that her husband has been sexual with every one of her close friends cancels travel plans to visit her family because he might do it again. A husband seeks out his wife's latest lover in an effort to stop their relationship. A wife buys her husband marijuana, which she hates to do, but rationalizes that it is better to have him numb on the couch than out exposing himself or chasing another woman. These people have in common the belief that it is in their power to stop the spouse's addiction. That is where their delusion begins, and as a result they become obsessed with their spouse's compulsive behavior. Ironically, efforts to control the spouse's behavior unwittingly intensify the addiction process.

Because our sexuality is one of our most fundamental life processes, sexual compulsiveness is extremely threatening to all of us. The intensity of our fears can be easily measured by the complex mosaic of proscriptions, laws, and taboos we use to guide our sexual behavior. This mosaic is the real expression of our values and cultural wisdom. When someone breaks a sexual taboo—in other words, goes beyond the socially acceptable limit—everyone's trust is shaken in our most fundamental social bonds, those "rules," written or commonly understood, that allow us as individuals to live comfortably with each other as a society.

While our society is shifting to a more open attitude toward sexual expression, we still view the amount and kind of activity as a matter of personal choice. For the addict, however, there is no choice. No choice. The addiction is in charge. That addicts have no control over their sexual behavior is a very hard concept to accept when the addicts' trails have left broken marriages and parentless children or, worse, victims of sexual crimes. Therefore, there are no neutral responses to sexual compulsivity.

Addicts, at one level, judge themselves by society's standards. Unable to measure up to these, they live with constant pain and alienation. Each one, convinced that he or she alone is afflicted, lives in isolation and constant fear of discovery. Addicts withhold a major portion of themselves—a pain deeply felt, but never expressed or witnessed. They do not trust nor do they become intimate with others, especially their families. There is the possibility that family members will find out about their behavior and the certainty that if that happens they would leave the addicts. As we shall see, fear of abandonment and shame are at the core of addiction. The alienation becomes a quagmire within which addicts struggle, only to become more isolated.

Family members, too, become more isolated as the addiction progresses. Their lives are filled with secret concerns about themselves and their families. Their worst fear is also discovery. What if what they suspect is true? What if something else happens? Spouses wonder about their attractiveness and sexuality, and they also fear abandonment and public ridicule. Children worry that the family problems are their fault. The sum total of the apprehension means that the family members end up feeling lonely, keeping secrets, and hurting. The obvious is ignored in the hopes it will disappear, and the family sinks deeper. Family members' efforts to struggle free also mire them even more quickly.

For both the addict and the family members, there is a way out. The Twelve Steps of Alcoholics Anonymous and Al-Anon have been a successful path to recovery for millions whose addiction was alcohol. The same process works for sexual addiction, providing a program by which one can live on a daily basis, short-circuiting that awful cycle in which what someone does to relieve pain makes him or her hurt even more. No longer do the sexual addicts and family members need to be alone with their illness. The Steps provide a process through which they can forgive themselves, make amends, and receive support for noncompulsive behavior.

If you are an addict or suspect you are and if you have the courage to face yourself, this book is intended for you. If you are a family member or concerned person, this book will also require courage and honesty, for it is about you as well. For the reader who, for whatever reason, finds it important to read this book, you too will have to struggle with your own beliefs and assumptions as you begin to appreciate our society's role in the addict's pain.

Ultimately, what is written here is about hope. By the reader's recognition of what happens in the addict's life, the isolation is, in fact, broken. The secret of the sexual addiction is out —people are not alone with the problem. Moreover, the Twelve Steps provide a concrete, proven path out of the quagmire.

In reading this book, there are some things to remember.

First, addiction taps into the most fundamental human processes. Whether the need is to be high, to be sexual, to eat, or even to work, the addictive process can turn creative, life-giving energy into a destructive, demoralizing compulsivity. The central losses are the addict's values and relationships. The phenomenon of multiple addictions is not surprising, given the pervasive nature of addiction. Overweight, over-work, and alcoholism are often part of the addict's life. So, in many ways, the book is a statement about the nature of addiction.

Also, the stories used in this book are fictionalized composites based on hundreds of First Step and Fourth Step preparations. They are carefully designed to be characterizations in order to protect individual anonymity. To the degree that they represent any individual is a comment on the commonality of the addicts' experiences. It may be even a greater indicator of how much we all—including nonaddicts—are part of the problem.

Please note: when I have chosen to use *he* and *him* as pronouns, it has been simply in order to preserve sentence continuity. This is with apology and full recognition to those women who have struggled so painfully with their addiction. Throughout the book, attention is given to the plight of women addicts. Their courage truly needs to be acknowledged.

For the professional who is looking for theoretical and empirical foundations, notes are collected for each chapter at the end of the book. For further information, look to the companion volume, *Contrary to Love: Helping the Sexual Addict* (Hazelden, 1989). In it is a history of how the concepts of sexual addiction were developed, including case histories, treatment planning, and intervention strategies. The issues in the companion book are of particular interest to counselors, judges, probation officers, and other professionals. Also, the resource guide at the back of this book provides lists of publications, Web sites, and professional societies relevant to this work.

This book is an effort to provide a nontechnical statement to help anyone—addicts, family members, and other concerned persons—to appreciate the nature and magnitude of the addict's problem and to discover how the Twelve Steps can be a path out of sexual compulsivity to recovery.

CHAPTER 1

The Addiction Cycle

◻ ◻ ◻

> Although Hefner was approaching forty-five, and had been in-
> volved with hundreds of photogenic women since starting his
> magazine, he enjoyed female companionship now more than
> ever; and perhaps more significant, considering all that Hefner
> had seen and done in recent years, was the fact that each occa-
> sion with a new woman was for him a novel experience. It was
> as if he was always watching for the first time a woman un-
> dress, rediscovering with delight the beauty of the female
> body, breathlessly expectant as panties were removed and
> smooth buttocks were exposed—and he never tired of the con-
> summate act. He was a sex junkie with an insatiable habit.
>
> —Gay Talese, *Thy Neighbor's Wife*

Del was a lawyer. Brilliant, charming, and witty. He had a
special breakthrough in his career when he was appointed as
one of the governor's special aides. His wife and three children were proud of his accomplishments. However, Del's
public visibility was creating a problem because he was also a
sexual addict. His double life included prostitution, porn
bookstores, and affairs.

Del would initiate relationships with women, feeling that he
was "in love." After the initial sexual contact, he would desperately wish to be free. These relationships became characterized

by his ambivalence. He wanted to be sexual, but he did not want the relationship. Yet he couldn't say no clearly without fear of hurting the women's feelings, so he never quite broke off the relationships. Instead he hoped their frustration would force them to give up. The result was that he had a series of relationships at the same time in various stages of initiation and frustration.

There was not only the juggling act of keeping his relationships straight. Some of these women were vital to him professionally. He exploited relationships to receive cooperation. His problem was that the women would believe that he cared for them. The professional complications were extreme. At one point, he was involved with a colleague and her secretary at the same time. The secretary went in to talk to her boss about this "problem" she had. Del had to face two very angry women.

His other behaviors were also problems. In porn shops, he was sexual with a number of men in the movie booths. Worse, the shops he frequented were near the capitol, an area where he was liable to be recognized. He vowed to stop when, sitting in a meeting in the attorney general's office, a plan was described for a raid on a local porn shop—the one he had patronized two days before. But he did not stop.

Neither were his visits to massage parlors without peril. One night his masseuse was a young girl quite high on some form of drug. Del decided to have his massage anyway, including a "hand job." When she masturbated him, she hurt his penis. Del was too shameful to complain or even to tell anybody. When he got home, he was so upset, he masturbated—despite his penis being sore.

Late one evening, Del pulled up next to a young woman at a stoplight. He had always had the fantasy of picking up a woman on a street. He looked at her and she smiled at him. Del became very excited. They drove side by side for several blocks. She returned his stares at each stop sign. Soon she pulled ahead of him, turned off the road, and pulled to a stop. He followed and pulled up behind her. She waved toward him and pulled out again. Del thought she wanted him to follow.

Del's mind raced ahead to where she could be leading him. She drove in the direction of a well-known local restaurant with a popular late-night bar. Convinced that was where they were headed, he speculated that after a drink, they might end up at her apartment. With his mind full of fantasies, he pulled up behind her when she stopped. As he was opening his door, she leaped out of her car and dashed into the building. Surprised, he looked up to see that he was not in front of the restaurant. Rather, she had stopped at the police station three blocks away.

Horrified, Del got back in his car and raced home. While driving, he was in shock at how out of touch with reality he was. She had not been encouraging him to follow her, but was in fact frightened. He, on the other hand, was so caught up in his fantasy that he failed to notice she was parking at a police station.

He felt a flood of remorse for subjecting the woman to a frightening ordeal. Also, he was terrified that she would accuse him of attempted rape and that he would be arrested. When Del arrived home at 1:30 A.M., he was so scared that he sat and prayed. At 2:00, there was a sound of a siren in the distance. He promised God that he would change. He fantasized about what it would do to his wife and kids. Truly, it was the most desperate moment of his life. Finally, he went to bed.

When he awoke in the morning, he felt tremendous relief. He knew he was not going to be picked up. He went to work and put enormous energy into his job that day. At the end of the day, he felt in need of a reward. He stopped at a massage parlor.

Del was a man who valued the law. He also prided himself

on his honesty with people, a fact he often parlayed into seduction. His children and wife were central to his life. He had
worked hard in his career. His addiction, however, violated his
own values and the law and jeopardized his career and family.
His story—of which just a few pieces are related here—is one
of constant predicaments. Del's addictive behavior put him in
situations in which he was vulnerable to tremendous consequences. His degradation was only exceeded by the violation
of his own principles. Because of Del's sexual addiction, his
fantasy became more real than the nightmare he created.

WHAT IS SEXUAL ADDICTION?

A way to understand sexual addicts like Del is to compare
them with other types of addicts. A common definition of
alcoholism or drug dependency is that a person has a pathological relationship with a mood-altering chemical.[1] The alcoholic's relationship with alcohol becomes more important
than family, friends, and work. The relationship progresses to
the point where alcohol is necessary to feel normal. To feel
"normal" for the alcoholic is also to feel isolated and lonely,
since the primary relationship he depends upon to feel adequate is with a chemical, not other people.

Sexual addiction is parallel. The addict substitutes a sick
relationship to an event or a process for a healthy relationship
with others. The addict's relationship with a mood-altering
experience becomes central to his life. Del, for example,
routinely jeopardized all that he loved. His vows to quit were
lost against the power of his addiction. The only thing that
exceeded his pain was his loneliness.

Addicts progressively go through stages in which they
retreat further from the reality of friends, family, and work.

Their secret lives become more real than their public lives. What other people know is a false identity. Only the individual addict knows the shame of living a double life—the real world and the addict's world.

Leading a fantasy double life is a distortion of reality. Del was so caught up in his fantasy that police station became a restaurant and a cooperative prospect was, in fact, a desperate and frightened woman. An essential part of sanity is being grounded in reality, so in the sense that addicts distort reality, the sexual addiction becomes a form of insanity.

THE ADDICT'S BELIEF SYSTEM

How does addiction begin? How does the progressive insanity occur? It begins with the delusional thought processes that are rooted in the addict's *belief system*. That is, addicts begin with core beliefs about themselves that affect how they perceive reality. So important is this factor—the belief system—in the addiction equation that it is a theme running throughout this entire book. For now, we need only to point out its role in the impaired thinking of the addict.

Each person has a belief system that is the sum of the assumptions, judgments, and myths that he or she holds to be true. It contains potent family messages about a person's value or worth, relationships, needs, and sexuality. Within it is a repertoire of what "options"—answers, solutions, methods, possibilities, ways of behaving—are open to each of us. In short, it is a model of the world.

On the basis of that model we

- plan and make decisions
- interpret other people's actions

- make meaning out of life experiences
- solve problems
- pattern our relationships
- develop our careers
- establish priorities

For each of us, our belief system is the filter through which we conduct the main task of our lives: making choices.

The addict's belief system contains certain core beliefs that are faulty or inaccurate and, consequently, that provide a fundamental momentum for the addiction. Generally, addicts do not perceive themselves as worthwhile persons. Nor do they believe that other people would care for them or meet their needs if everything was known about them, including the addiction. Finally, they believe that sex is their most important need. Sex is what makes isolation bearable. Their core beliefs are the anchor points of the sexual addiction. If you do not trust people, one thing that is true about sex—and alcohol, food, gambling, and risk—is that it always does what it promises—for the moment. Thus, as in our definition of addiction, the relationship is with sex—and not people.

Impaired Thinking

Out of the belief system—the set of interacting faulty beliefs—come distorted views of reality. Denial leads the list of ways that addicts distort reality. Addicts use many devices to deny—to themselves and others—that there is a problem. Ignoring the problem, blaming others, and minimizing the behaviors are part of the addict's defensive repertoire. Consequences such as venereal disease, unwanted pregnancy, lost jobs, arrests, and broken relationships are either overlooked or attributed to factors other than the addiction:

- Venereal disease: "A lot of people get it now."
- Pregnancy: "She tricked me into it."
- Arrests: "Cops had it in for me. They had no real proof."
- Jobs: "The boss needs to be liberated."
- Relationships: "Her family always had problems. She simply couldn't handle it."

When addicts believe in the defensive rationalizations, the result is *denial* that a specific incident or behavior is a part of a total behavioral pattern.

Arguments, excuses, justifications, and circular reasoning abound in the addict's impaired mental processes:

- If I don't have it every few days, the pressure builds up.
- I am oversexed and have to meet my needs.
- What she doesn't know won't hurt.
- My husband is not sensitive to my needs.
- She really enjoyed, asked for, deserved it.
- Only certain men turn me on, and my husband isn't one of them.
- Every guy will get what "nookie" he can.
- If only my wife would be more responsive.
- Men are like animals—males are more sexual than females.
- Cybersex is just electrons; it's not real.
- With the stress I am under, I deserve it.
- It doesn't hurt anybody because . . .
- The Internet helps to broaden my sexual horizons.
- I couldn't help it, given how she acted.
- No one really cares.
- It's my way of relaxing.
- Internet chat rooms don't hurt anybody—it's just a game.
- Women always pretend they don't want it when they do.

Whatever the *rationalization*, it further cuts the addict off from the reality of his or her behavior.

Sincere delusion is believing your own lies. The addicts who make a commitment to change or follow through on something are sincere in their intentions. They are as sincere as when they vow to themselves to quit. They may even experience a great deal of emotion—tears of pain, expressions of tenderness, or anger when someone doesn't believe in their good intentions. However, their commitment to others is no more valid than their vows to themselves. It might seem paradoxical to be sincere about telling a lie. It is not, but it is evidence of seriously impaired thinking.

An example of the thinking process will help. The addict who has been confronted by his wife because he was not at work when he was supposed to be spins out a tale as to his whereabouts. She doubts he is telling the truth. He is incensed at her distrust. He assumes she would be this way even if he were truthful. So he takes it a step further. He assures her that he had even told her earlier that he'd be where he now says he was. This makes her feel even crazier, because she cannot remember. His emotions about her distrust are real. He is now even more incensed that she cannot remember. His lies and his sincerity become fused.

Making declarations of love in order to seduce, becoming incensed at the behavior of an arresting officer in order to obscure one's own behavior, and protesting that something "happened only once" in order to cover up—all are types of sincere delusion.

Ironically, the addict knows that he really is *not* trustworthy. In his isolation, he is also convinced that most people cannot be trusted. Further, he is certain that if anyone found out about his secret life of addictive experiences, there would be no forgiveness. Only judgment. To complicate matters, he has placed himself in so many precarious situations that he lives in constant fear of discovery of his being so untrustworthy. The *suspicion* and *paranoia* heighten the sense of alienation.

The addict's blame of others for all problems is another way to protect his secret life. Fault lies with spouse, children, parents, work associates, or boss. The addict is self-righteous, critical, and judgmental. There is no acceptance of personal responsibility for mistakes, failures, or actions. This appearance of integrity further insulates the addict's world from reality. The *blame dynamic* provides further justification for the addict's behavior. Ungrateful children, demanding spouses, hard-nosed bosses create an unfair world in which the addict deserves a reward. To be honest about one's limitations would bring the wall crumbling down—and, in turn, jeopardize the one source of nurturing and care that can be counted on: the sexual addiction.

Each of these delusional thought processes—denial, rationalization, sincere delusion, paranoia, and blame—closes off an important avenue of self-knowledge and touch with reality for the addict. Gone are the feedback loops that serve as vital correctives to a faulty belief system. In this way the addict's world becomes closed off from the real world. Within that world the addictive cycle is now free to work.

THE ADDICTION CYCLE

For sexual addicts an addictive experience progresses through a four-step cycle that intensifies with each repetition:

1. *Preoccupation*—the trance or mood wherein the addicts' minds are completely engrossed with thoughts of sex. This mental state creates an obsessive search for sexual stimulation.

2. *Ritualization*—the addicts' own special routines that lead up to the sexual behavior. The ritual intensifies the preoccupation, adding arousal and excitement.
3. *Compulsive sexual behavior*—the actual sexual act, which is the end goal of the preoccupation and ritualization. Sexual addicts are unable to control or stop this behavior.
4. *Despair*—the feeling of utter hopelessness addicts have about their behavior and their powerlessness.

The pain the addicts feel at the end of the cycle can be numbed or obscured by sexual preoccupation that reengages the addiction cycle.

Sexual addicts are hostages of their own *preoccupation*. Every passerby, every relationship, and every introduction to someone passes through the sexually obsessive filter. More than merely noticing sexually attractive people, there is a quality of desperation that interferes with work, relaxation, and even sleep. People become objects to be scrutinized. A walk through a crowded downtown area is translated into a veritable shopping list of "possibilities."

To understand the trancelike state of preoccupation, imagine the intense passion of courtship. We laugh at two lovers who are so absorbed in one another that they forget about their surroundings. The *intoxication* of young love is what the addict attempts to capture. It is the pursuit, the hunt, the search, the suspense heightened by the unusual, the stolen, the forbidden, the illicit that are intoxicating to the sexual addict. The new conquest of the hustler; the score of the exposer, voyeur, or rapist; or the temptation of breaking the taboo of sex with one's child—in essence, they are variations of a theme: courtship gone awry. Nowhere is this more visible than in the search for sex on the Internet. Hours pass while you're gazing at pornographic images on the computer screen or sending instant messages. There is total preoccupation. You might find yourself not sleeping because you're tranced in cyberspace. You might not be working during the day because you're too exhausted and you feel compelled to go online for sex despite promising yourself you wouldn't. Progressively, your relationships suffer. Kids are neglected. Spouses are ignored. Phone calls remain unreturned. Isolation becomes real.

The addict uses—or abuses, rather—one of the most exciting moments in human experience: sex. Sexual arousal becomes intensified. The addict's mood is altered as he enters the obsessive trance. The metabolic responses are like a rush through the body as androgens speed up the body's functioning. The heart pounds as the addict focuses on his search object. Risk, danger, and even violence are the ultimate escalators. One can always increase the dosage of intoxication. Preoccupation effectively buries the personal pain of remorse or regret. The addict does not always have to act. Often just thinking about acting brings relief.

The sexual addict's excitement-seeking parallels some other types of compulsive/obsessive addicts. In that sense, there is little difference between the voyeur waiting for hours by a window for ninety seconds of nudity and the compulsive gambler hunching on a long shot. What makes the sexual addict different is that he draws upon the human emotions generated by courtship and passion.

The trance is enhanced by the sexual addict's *ritualization*. Professionals have often wondered why sex offenders use the same "MO" (modus operandi or method) each time, when it only makes apprehension easier. The answer is simple. A ritual helps the trance. Like a yogi in meditation, the addict does not have to stop and think or disrupt his focus. The ritual itself, like preoccupation, can start the rush of excitement.

Addicts often talk about their rituals. The compulsive

masturbator and his surroundings, the incestuous father and his elaborate preparations, the cybersex addict and starting the modem, the exposer's regular routes, the hustler's approach and cruising area—all involve complex rituals. The rituals contain a set of well-rehearsed cues that trigger arousal.

The preoccupation trance supported by extensive rituals is as important as—or sometimes more important than—sexual contact or orgasm. The intoxication of the whole experience is what the addict seeks in order to move through the cycle from despair to exhilaration. One cannot be orgasmic all the time. So the search and the suspense absorb the addict's concentration and energy. Cruising, watching, waiting, preparing are part of the mood alteration.

The first two phases of the addictive cycle (preoccupation and ritualization) are not always visible. The addict struggles to present an image of normalcy to the outside world. The public self is a false ego, since the addict knows the incongruity of his double life. Compulsive sexual behavior, the third phase of the cycle, however, leaves a trail, despite the protective public image.

In the story of Del, described earlier in this chapter, he repeatedly made commitments to himself and to God that he would stop. These resolves were short-lived. Del could not control his behavior even though he wanted to. Like Del, addicts are *powerless* over their behavior. They have lost control over their sexual expression, which is exactly why they are defined as *addicts*. The failure of their efforts to control their behavior is a sign of their addiction. Sexual addicts often describe the process of picking a day—a child's birthday, a change of jobs, a holiday—as "the last day." Usually, this marks a time when "it" will never happen again. Sometimes addicts will set goals—a year, a month, or a week. Whether forever or a shorter time, the addicts betray themselves, buying into the delusion that they are in control of their behavior. When they fail, yet another indictment of self-control and morality is added to ever-increasing shame. For the recovering addicts who have acknowledged powerlessness, there is hope. They know that they might get through one day free from their addiction—with a lot of help.

The *despair* that the addict experiences after being compulsively sexual is the "low" phase of the four-step cycle. The letdown combines the sense of failure at not having lived up to resolutions to stop with hopelessness about ever being able to stop. If the behavior was particularly degrading, humiliating, or risky, the addict's self-pity grows. If the behavior violated basic personal values or exploited them, the addict experiences self-hatred as well. Addicts often report suicidal feelings along with their despair and shame.

Standing in the wings, however, is the ever-ready preoccupation that can pull the addict out of the doldrums. The cycle then becomes self-perpetuating. Each repetition builds upon the previous experiences and solidifies the reiterative pattern of the addiction. As the cycle fastens its grip on the addict, the addict's life starts to disintegrate and become unmanageable.

Unmanageability

The addict is caught up in the task of keeping his secret life from affecting his "public" life. Even so, the consequences come: arrests, unmasked lies, disruption, unmet commitments, attempts to explain the unexplainable. The addiction surfaces in the addict's inability to manage his life. For a moment, the addict recognizes that he cannot continue. But the impaired mental process blurs reality with euphoric recall of sexual successes. The addict faces yet again the ultimate seduction: a unique opportunity that, of course, will be "the last time."

This unending struggle to manage two lives—"normal" and addictive—continues. The unmanageability takes its toll. Family and friendships are abbreviated and sacrificed. Hobbies are neglected. Finances are affected. Physical needs of other kinds are unattended. The addict's lifestyle becomes a consistent violation of his or her own values, compounding the shame. The impaired mental processes result in faulty problem solving in all areas of the addict's life. These decisions add to further unmanageability.

Nowhere is this more clear than in the workplace. Faulty problem solving and diversion of energy require extra time and effort to hold down the job. Extra long hours at work further the unmanageability at home. Worse, if the addiction is connected with the work environment, the addict's position is even more precarious.

Addicts often point to the connection between their addiction and the stress of high performance demands in which there is important personal investment. Graduate school, for example, is often when addicts first encounter compulsiveness. The stress of proving one's self in an arena where every inadequacy is evaluated is a potent flash point for the ignition of sexual addiction. So are new jobs, promotions, and solo business ventures. Unstructured time, a heavy responsibility for self-direction, and high demands for excellence seem to be the common elements in these situations that are easy triggers for addictive behaviors. Procrastination becomes a daily nemesis for these addicts. For once ignited, the addiction makes work easy to put off.

One of the worst consequences of the addiction is the addicts' *isolation*. The intensity of the double life relates directly to the distance of the addicts from their friends and families. That is, the more intensely involved in compulsive sexual life the addicts become, the more alienated they become from their parents, spouses, and children. Without those human connections, the addicts paradoxically lose touch with their own selves. The unmanageability from the addiction has run its course when there is no longer a double life. When there are no longer friends or family to protect or a job to hold or pretenses to be made—even though some things are valued enough to want to stop—the addiction is at its most destructive and violent point. The addict's world has become totally insulated from real life.

THE ADDICTIVE SYSTEM

As addicts move from healthy relationships to sexual compulsion, their internal processes combine to form an addictive system. The addictive system—as with all systems—contains subsystems that support one another. Often this support occurs in repetitive, predictable cycles.

To picture the addictive system with its subsystems, consider the human body. It is a complex system with many subsystems—the nervous system, the digestive system, and so on. Clearly, when one subsystem, such as the nervous system, is upset, all the other bodily systems are affected and must adjust in some way.

The addictive system starts with a belief system containing faulty assumptions, myths, and values that support impaired thinking. The resulting delusional thought processes insulate the addiction cycle from reality. The four-phase addiction cycle (preoccupation, ritualization, sexual compulsiveness, and despair) can repeat itself unhindered and take over the addict's life. All the other support systems, including relationships, work, finance, and health, become unmanageable. The negative consequences from the unmanageability confirm the faulty beliefs, which hold that the addict is a bad person who is unlovable. In turn, revalidated beliefs allow further distortion of reality. Diagrammed, the addictive system looks like this:

THE ADDICTIVE SYSTEM

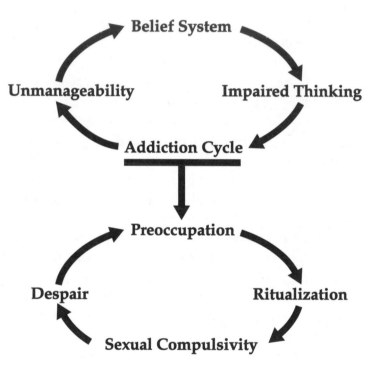

Figure 1.1

Within the addictive system, *sexual experience becomes the reason for being—the primary relationship for the addict.* For the addict, the sexual experience is the source of nurturing, focus of energy, and origin of excitement. It is the remedy for pain and anxiety, the reward for success, and the means for maintaining emotional balance. Outsiders, especially those who care about the addict, witness the unmanageability and maybe even the behavior. They see the addict's personal loss, the self-degradation, and the abandoned hope and values. It would seem so simple to just stop—even for a while. For the exhibitionist, for example, who may spend up to seven hours a day cruising and another four thinking about it, the task is not so easy. The addiction is truly an altered state of consciousness in which "normal" sexual behavior pales by comparison in terms of excitement and relief from troubles.

In the addict's world, there is an ongoing tension between a person's normal self and the addicted self. A Jekyll/Hyde struggle emerges. The addictive system is so compelling that to stop would be like death. Yet, as the system continues, the person's values, priorities, and loved ones are attacked. Sometimes, only a major crisis can restore perspective. Such was the case of Carrie.

Carrie was a music teacher. She was known for boundless energy and creativity in music. She served four elementary schools, carrying heavy equipment from school to school in her old red Volkswagen bus. The kids loved her and she loved them. Colleagues admired her skills. Parents were grateful and attended her concerts in masses.

Carrie had another life as well. Her singing was true and compelling. She received regular engagements at local nightspots. She dreamed of being a star. Her singing career, however, never got beyond the local piano bar circuit. No matter how hard she tried, her professional singing career was stymied. As she approached the age of thirty, her disappointment grew into panic that her dream might not happen.

Carrie's sexual addiction started to flourish at the point when she began panicking about her career. In the beginning there were occasional one-night stands with hotel customers in bars in which she sang. Then it became every night she worked. The ritual started with her looking over the patrons, selecting the most interesting. Animated conversations during the breaks followed. After finishing, she would go to his room and have sex. Leaving at three or four in the morning, she would return home for a few hours of sleep before school started.

She did not like what she was doing. In the morning, looking at the trusting faces of the children, she would feel the profound incongruity of where she had been but a few hours before. Also, her teaching was slipping as the addiction progressed, though no one really noticed but her. The children were still excited and everyone she worked with was convinced she was great. Still, she knew. She even discovered that being at four different schools made it easier for her to cover when she overslept. She had simply "stopped at one of the other schools."

Carrie had also ceased dating and started singing on weekends. Since she lived alone, her only human contacts were the children and her piano bar customers. What she really wanted was a husband and a family. As her addiction progressed, she began to believe no man would want to be with her if he knew about her life.

The consequence that brought Carrie help was an unexpected heart attack at the age of thirty-three. The short nights had taken their toll. Finally, sitting in a hospital bed, Carrie told her story to a woman chaplain. Amid deep sobs, she talked of her loneliness and her love of the children. Through her conversations with the chaplain, Carrie acknowledged that the number of men she had slept with in the three-year period was in the hundreds. It was a miracle she had not contracted venereal disease or HIV/AIDS or been injured or even murdered. The damage to her self-image was devastating enough.

Carrie, like all sexual addicts, lived in two worlds. One was a world of piano bars, musty hotel rooms, and nameless faces. The other had music, laughter, and faces of children and colleagues—whose names she knew. The coexistence of the two worlds continued until Carrie's body refused to live up to the strain.

OTHER ADDICTIONS AND EMOTIONAL ILLNESS

One other aspect of the addictive system is that the belief system and delusional thought patterns may support more than one addiction. Overeating, for example, is a way to minimize pain. The sexual addicts who become overweight add shame concerning their body image to their repertoire of pain. The two addictions start to reinforce each other. When the addicts believe that people are not attracted to them, their sexual addiction is partially rooted in the fear of rejection. Then they eat compulsively to kill the pain due to the fear of rejection, and as a result put on weight. The added weight, by their standards, makes them even less desirable. Also, one way to avoid the depression after sexually bingeing is to binge again—with food. The two processes become interdependent. Addicts who have both addictions report that at the height of their sexual addiction, they had their greatest weight problem. We know that 38 percent of sex addicts also struggle with an eating disorder.[2]

By far the most common combination of addictions is when the sexual addict is also dependent on alcohol or another drug. Many people attribute sexual excesses and even incest to the power of alcoholism. *The reality is that alcoholism often is a concurrent illness with, rather than the cause of, the sexual addiction.*

Many alcoholics have discovered that the treatment of one addiction does not cure the other. Further, many discover that they drink or use to obliterate the pain of their sexual behavior. There is a growing documentation about the interaction between the two addictions.[3] In fact, we know that 42 percent of sex addicts have a problem with chemical dependency.[4] Among cocaine addicts, 50 to 70 percent have a problem with sexual compulsion.[5] It may be that one of the greatest, unacknowledged contributors to recidivism in alcoholism is the failure of treatment programs to treat multiple addictions.

All types of compulsive behavior may be woven into the scenario of sexual addiction.[6] Shoplifting, gambling, and spending are frequent counterparts. Physical violence as a way to release pent-up tension is often reported as a concurrent behavior by sexually abusive families. The workaholic who gets high on the excitement of a new achievement finds professional life even more exhilarating when coupled with the sexual addiction. In that case, the sexual and work addict marries the job. In a pool of thousands of sex addicts, fewer than 13 percent reported having just one addiction.

Emotional illness also flourishes within the addict's world. Depression, bipolar disorders, suicide, obsessive-compulsive behavior, and post-traumatic stress disorder are frequent companions to the addiction. Many addicts have received treatment for these mental illnesses while the concomitant sexual addiction is ignored. Yet the sexual addiction compounded the mental health issues. By far the most devastating emotional risk is suicide.[7] Seventeen percent of sex addicts have attempted suicide; 72 percent have thought of it. To preserve his integrity, Dr. Jekyll had to kill Mr. Hyde. Some sexual addicts become so desperate during the fourth phase of the addiction cycle (the despair after the compulsive behavior) that the only way out of the double life they can see is to die. Like Dr. Jekyll, sexual addicts' suicidal and depressed feelings express the powerlessness and impotence of living in the addicts' world.

RECOVERY

Recovery from addiction is the reversal of the alienation that is integral to the addiction. Addicts must establish roots in a caring community. With that support, addicts can stay straight as they struggle for a perspective on their lives. With help, addicts can integrate new beliefs and discard dysfunctional thinking. Without the mood-altering insanity to insulate them from knowledge about their own selves, they become participants in the restoration of their own sanity.

All forms of addiction are vicious because they further the inability to trust others. Yet without help from others, the addict cannot regain control because the addiction feeds itself. The sexual addiction is especially virulent because few forms of fixation or excitement are as supercharged with social judgment, ridicule, or fear. Consequently, seeking help is especially difficult for the sexual addict.

One of the best-proven paths to recovery is the Twelve Steps of Alcoholics Anonymous.[8] Many people suffering from compulsive disorders have translated the Steps for their own use, such as Overeaters Anonymous, Gamblers Anonymous, and Emotions Anonymous. This book proposes the Twelve Steps as a way for sexual addicts to emerge from their double lives. Across the country local groups have modified the Twelve Steps for the sexually compulsive. They go by names such as Sex and Love Addicts Anonymous, Sex Addicts Anonymous, Sexaholics Anonymous, or Sexual Compulsives Anonymous.

These Twelve Step programs help members restore the living network of human relationships—especially in the family. Step One asks the addicts first to accept their addiction by looking at their addiction cycle and its consequences, that is, to admit that they are powerless over their sexual behavior and their lives have become unmanageable. With that admission, the members then are able to start the rebuilding of relationships by taking responsibility for what they have done and making amends where possible. Values and priorities are reclaimed. Throughout the program, members explore basic spiritual issues as a way of understanding and facing their anxiety. As members live the program, the double life, with all its delusion and pain, can be left behind. Chapter 7 of this book describes in detail how the Twelve Steps can help the sexual addict break out of the addicts' world.

This chapter has described the cycle of sexual addiction. Before proceeding further, we must survey the many forms sexual addiction can take. No assessment of the sexual addiction would be complete without showing its potential variations. The question to be answered is, Who are the inhabitants of the addicts' world? That is the task of the next chapter.

CHAPTER 2

The Levels of Addiction

◼   ◼   ◼

Herb, 34, is a traveling salesman who maintains an apartment in Minneapolis for his regular visits to the city. He is married and has two children. He earns about $35,000 a year. Herb says he has a good relationship with his wife of seven years, but that spending nearly half of his life on the road drives him to prostitutes.

At the same time, he admits that he probably would continue to visit prostitutes—although not as frequently—even if his work did not keep him away from home so much.

Herb said he has been patronizing prostitutes for nine years and seeks encounters on an average of two or three times a week when he is not at home.

"I think of them as therapy," Herb said, "and I'm serious now. I usually go during the middle of the day, and it's often when something's bugging me. I've had a bad morning or a sale has gone sour.

"Instead of going out to lunch and downing two or three martinis, I like to have a woman."

—*Minneapolis Star*, October 7, 1976

We live in a time where the "joy of sex" is seen as the rightful pursuit of everyone. To be celibate, in fact, is almost to be suspect. As part of the sexual revolution, inhibitions and hang-ups are to be discarded. In many ways, this shift in our cultural mores constitutes a breakthrough in the exploration of human sexuality. It is an important antidote to the proscriptive past and a significant acknowledgment of our sexual nature. As in all major culture changes, there are excesses. Our preoccupation with sex pervades almost all facets of our contemporary lifestyles. In an age that highly values the variety and quality of sexual experience, there is a group that is overlooked: those who are sexually compulsive in ways they do not want to be.

To view sexual addicts as people who are simply guilt-ridden because of sexual behavior is to completely misunderstand the nature of the addiction. This viewpoint assumes that addicts need to be more free and enjoy sexuality and that they feel bad because of unhelpful scruples and misinformation. An example is masturbation, which is now generally accepted as a developmental phase and a natural expression of personal sexuality. For the man who masturbates so often that he has at times severely injured his penis, it is no longer just a question of accepting his desire to masturbate. His masturbation is seriously affecting his life and bringing harmful consequences to his body.

Sexual addicts feel the pain and consequences. They recognize the personal emptiness. If they are lucky, they may have some sense of the exploitation and harm to others. They wrestle daily with the fear of discovery of their compulsivity. This is not to suggest that sexual addicts are uninhibited and free of hang-ups. On the contrary, they often do come from highly repressive families and carry damaging myths inside them. Part of recovery is always restructuring the belief system by acquiring adequate information and accepting one's own sexuality. The first task of recovery, however, is to focus on the uncontrollable behavior.

When discussing sexual addiction, it is necessary to recognize that not everyone who has a regrettable sexual experience is an addict. There are people who have regrets over specific events, realizing that their sexual behavior on a given occasion was not in their best interest. They add it to their experience and simply do not repeat it. There are numbers of people who have occasionally abused their sexuality. Going on a sexual binge, for example, might occur after a graduation or in retaliation to a lover's indiscretion.

There are also those who have episodes of compulsivity. Those who study middle-age transition, the famous "middlescence," note the sexual bingeing that can occur at that time. It is also often seen as a postdivorce pattern. The divorced person, who is suddenly free from marital obligations, may experiment to excess. Adolescents struggle with the intensity of their emerging sexuality. Adolescent sexual expression is a key conflict area between peer support and parental proscription. Experimentation and exploration are part of identity formation. Learning from youthful enthusiasm is part of internalizing appropriate rules and boundaries. In that sense, adolescence does parallel the "middlescence" search for self. Thus, episodes of sexual excess may only indicate changing life circumstances.[1]

Also, there are those who may have a problem, but not necessarily an addiction. Consider the story of Don, a college professor nationally recognized for his careful scholarship. On occasion he had the urge to go to a porn theater. While watching the movie, he would masturbate, which he found very exciting. When leaving, however, an immense depression would always come over him. He felt degraded. He worried about being recognized—or worse—arrested. He would always vow not to repeat the experience. Over a period of eight years, he had done it four to five times.

Don's problem has some important parallels with sexual addiction. The excitement/depression scenario is a common story for the addict. So are breaking the rules and the excitement of the illicit. Also, the vow to quit or make it the last time is part and parcel of the addiction. Yet Don is not an addict. This is not to minimize his problem, which is painful and abusive. He runs the risk of adverse consequences, but, in general, his life has not become unmanageable. In short, he has not entered the addict's world. Were Don to experience periods in which he repeated the behavior frequently with damaging results, he clearly would have an addictive pattern. Many addicts describe their experiences as episodic—that is, they occur in periodic binges that have severe consequences to their work, relationships, and self-esteem. Between binges, they may experience extended periods with no problems. Being able to stop for a period of time provides the illusion of control, which makes it more difficult for the addict to acknowledge that there is a problem. As years pass, however, a pattern of bingeing reveals an unmistakable addiction. For some addicts, the bingeing becomes so frequent that the behavior is almost constant.

If Don's situation were changed again and his visits to the theater were a part of a much larger picture, including massage parlors, strip shows, and multiple affairs, his actions also would have a very different meaning. A clear case of addiction can emerge when other forms of sexual compulsiveness are considered as well. The assessment of the addiction's extent or intensity is not complete without first examining the varieties of sexual addiction.

LEVELS OF ADDICTION

Addicts often comment in group therapy that they are astounded at how similar their experiences were, even though what they did was vastly different. While the varieties of addiction are great, the sexual addiction cycle described in chapter 1 is common. Categorizing the various forms of sexual compulsiveness into different groups, however, helps in a number of ways. First, grouping provides perspective on the wide range of sexual behaviors in which addiction can thrive. From this perspective addicts can make a better inventory of the scope of their addiction. Second, some sexual behavior involves great danger, breaks the law, or victimizes others. For the addicts, these behaviors show greater powerlessness and unmanageability. To risk greater consequences in the interest of a more exciting high indicates the *escalation of the addiction*. Finally, every addict must understand his or her own unique pattern of sexually compulsive behavior. Subtle differences are extremely important for addicts, especially in early recovery. For example, strategies for avoiding unique cues and rituals that initiate the addictive cycle can be developed once a pattern is identified. To interrupt the addictive cycle the addict must understand his or her pattern of behavior. Creating a framework for the behavior has made that task easier.

A workable structure that helps to identify patterns is to view the addiction as operating at three levels. Level One contains behaviors that are regarded as normal, acceptable, or tolerable. Examples include masturbation, pornography, and prostitution. Level Two, by contrast, extends to those behaviors which are clearly victimizing and for which legal sanctions are enforced. These are generally seen as nuisance offenses, such as exhibitionism or voyeurism. The Level Three behaviors have grave consequences for the victims and legal consequences for the addicts; examples are incest, child molestation, or rape. Compulsivity at this level represents a severe progression of the addiction.

Suggesting three levels does not mean that addicts cannot destroy their lives with Level One behavior. Many addicts have done just that without ever venturing into Levels Two or Three. It would be unusual, however, for an addict to be compulsive at Levels Two or Three without a significant amount of compulsivity at Level One. Most rare is the addict who simply focuses on only one form of sexual compulsiveness. But that, too, does happen. Within a level or across levels, the addict must understand the full range of possibilities.

Some people have considered the levels as really a sign of progression—that is, addicts start at Level One and inevitably end up at Level Three. Or they consider that the potential is there. Actually, the vast majority of addicts are at Levels One and Two. Many sex offenders do not fit the criteria for addiction. So offending behavior does not equal addictive behavior. Addiction results when the offenses are either embedded in a wide pattern of behaviors or the offending behaviors themselves are compulsive. Finally, some addicts start at Level Three and then focus only on Level One behaviors. The levels simply help us organize potentially addictive behaviors by how the culture views them.

Level One

Level One behaviors have in common general cultural acceptance. If some are regarded as unseemly or even illegal, the reality is that widespread practice conveys a public tolerance. The other common characteristic is that each can be devastating when done compulsively. Even the healthiest forms of human sexual expression can turn into self-defeating behaviors—or worse—the victimization of others.

Masturbation

Masturbation is an essential part of being a sexual person. Nurturing oneself, exploring sexual needs and fantasies, and establishing a basic self-knowledge are vital contributions that masturbation makes to sexual identity. As sexual therapists are keenly aware, without these factors it is more difficult to have a vital sexual relationship. In fact, for people who suffer from sexual dysfunction, therapy often involves a careful rebuilding of a patient's attitudes and beliefs around masturbation.

For the addict, however, masturbation becomes a degrading event. Masturbating four to five times a day for years on end becomes a secret life. It is the central part of every day. At the least feeling of frustration or loneliness, the addict struggles to find a private place to masturbate. Unlocking the office door, walking out of the bathroom, or driving in the car, addicts are certain that no one else is as obsessed as they are.

Part of that certainty comes from the collection of judgments and beliefs they hold to be true about masturbation. Messages from parents, family, and church have left no doubt that it is a character flaw. As a result, addicts may carry some equation in their head: Masturbation equals failure. Masturbation equals a loss of manhood. Masturbation is not feminine. Masturbation equals punishment.

One addict tells a story about his Catholic upbringing. Each Saturday, his father would ask if the boy had to go to confession. Since masturbation was a sin, both boy and father knew what had to be confessed. The father would talk to the boy about how he would become a man when he conquered his urges. The boy would sit in his shame. He dreaded Saturdays.

It later turned out that the father was simply telling his own belief, his own myth, to the boy. The father was a compulsive masturbator who believed that his problem was simply lack of self-control. In his desperation to prevent the same pain for his son, the father relayed the myth that locked him into his own addiction. (The same image of ideal manliness that added to the father's shame was passed on to his son.) Paradoxically, he recreated the same addictive system for his son out of love. As addicts go, this is a common story.

The son translated the message in a particularly damaging way. He felt that God would punish him for his masturbation. In fact, he believed that nothing would go right for him for the twenty-four hours following each time he masturbated. Given the power of his expectations and his daily masturbation, his life was an unending cycle of failure and disappointments. His compulsive masturbating was central to the self-fulfilling prophecy of God's punishment.

Compulsive Relationships

Addiction can manifest itself in a relationship in a number of ways. At the most elementary level, addiction is present when one partner sacrifices important parts of the total relationship in the service of sexual needs. A warning sign is when a spouse or significant other starts to feel victimized by the other's sexuality. (The warning intensifies when exploited feelings are dismissed.) Discounting the partner's feelings trades relationship needs for sexual needs. Every relationship has times when sexual needs are not matched. The addict, however, makes the other person an obsession. For the partner, the relationship is contingent on sexual performance. Both partners lose the freedom, fun, and intimacy of mutual loving sexual play. Sexuality ceases to be nurturing, growing, and life-enhancing. Addiction renders a relationship empty, joyless, and demoralizing.

Some addicts seek refuge in multiple relationships. Consider the woman whose loneliness is enhanced by an unending series of one-night stands. Try as she will, she cannot stop the blur of faces and bodies. Or take the man who seldom has one relationship but is "meaningfully" involved with several simultaneously. When he stops to be honest, he may admit not even liking his sexual partners. To have perceived the relationships as meaningful was a delusion used to get them into bed. The human dilemma of whether it is possible to love more than one person at once is not what is in question. At issue here is the fear of having to live without sex. Or, in addiction terms, the addict must protect the supply.

The Internet appears to be the ultimate experience for the romance junkie. Since it is often seen as only "electrons" and not real, addicts can rationalize that Web romancing is really not being unfaithful, in much the same way that a "virtual" game is not real. E-mails, instant messaging, and chat rooms become the outlets for all the unresolved intimacy, abandonment, and loneliness issues. Romance junkies fail to realize all the time it takes away from the real people in their lives.

Cruising is one of the ultimate activities for the desperate addict. Hustling in bars, streets, and parties is characterized by the contrast of excitement and loneliness. Will I be chosen? Will I score? Even the prospect is exhilarating. Memories of successful forays—the smells, the music, the adventures— cloak the sadness. The pursuit of sexual excitement extends to professional, business, and educational settings. However, the void that sex attempts to fill remains the same.

Chris, for example, was an addict whose cruising was fused with her professional life as a consultant in urban planning. Her ability to articulate clearly the complex problems of her field plus her charisma and attractiveness made her a speaker in high demand. Her life was filled with seminars, conferences, and workshops. They served as a cover for her other life. Her traveling maximized her sexual opportunities. She had ongoing relationships in each of the cities she visited regularly. One-night stands were even more common. With hindsight, she was later to say that to travel was to be sexual. It started as soon as she stepped on the plane. Her career was a potent catalyst to the addiction.

Cruising as a search for sexual excitement can even occur within the context of marriage, sometimes with tragic results. Fred and Liza were considered the ideal couple by their friends. Sweethearts at age fourteen and married at age twenty, their addiction problems started when both were in graduate school. Liza had come home one night after being at a bar and confessed to Fred that she had been picked up and "made." Fred's response was unexpected. He found it exciting and made ardent love to her. He asked her to do it again, with similar results. Soon their lovemaking became a ritual in which Liza would seduce a man, report all the details to Fred, and make love with Fred.

As the excitement grew old, Fred encouraged Liza to bring the men home. Fred would masturbate as he watched the men with his wife. Eventually, he took more of an active role in orchestrating the activities, which became progressively more degrading to Liza. After years, their married life was organized around these events. When they finally sought therapy, the striking part of their story was how each had longed to stop. They had even made mutual efforts to stop, especially after a time when Liza was injured. The central part of their recovery was in reclaiming their very real love of each other.

Centerfolds, Pornography, and Strip Shows

Playboy, Oui, Penthouse, Hustler, and other magazines are available online, at drugstores, grocery stores, and even the neighborhood "Quickstop." You can choose magazines for whatever your interest—gay, lesbian, barely legal, over fifty, African American, Asian, motorcycle, spring break, and leather. You can purchase or rent X-rated movies or trade home movies. Porn shops abound. Erotic art has been legitimized. The human body is a career focus for some of the best photographers. Many establishments feature topless and bottomless entertainment to bring in patrons. The more refined clubs use "lingerie" shows. The advent of cybersex and cable TV has added many new dimensions to offices, hotel rooms, porn shops, and even the bedroom. Nude beaches are no longer uncommon.

Some of the sexual art is creative, some is erotic, some reflects shifts in cultural boundaries. Some is titillating. Some is crass commercialism. Some is realism. Some is boring. Some is in bad taste.

Taken together, a veritable smorgasbord of obsession for the addict exists. One common element is the excitement. The other is the sexual object. The addict can transform even the most refined forms of human nudity into his own particular fusion of loneliness and arousal. The absence of a relationship and the desire for heightened excitement are the twin pillars of the sexual addiction. Nowhere is this more clear than when the addiction is visual.

Visual addiction does not always have obvious consequences. It is common to see men straining their necks as they drive, in order to watch an attractive woman walk down a street on a summer day. The addict, however, will turn around to go by her a second time—perhaps nearly causing an accident—in an effort to watch her again. An addict can spend endless hours browsing in a porn bookstore, cruising porn Web sites, sitting in the beach parking lot, driving around a college campus or a shopping mall, or stopping nightly at the topless bar. Soon the time takes its toll. Work does not get done and excuses are made. Lies are told to the family about the long work hours.

The lack of money starts to be an issue. For instance,

money needed for family expenses is spent on pornography, on computer sex in its myriad forms, and on sexually explicit CDs or videotapes. Then there is the camera equipment for a hobby not enjoyed except for the excitement of asking people to pose.

The worst is that after a time, the obsession becomes more significant than being in an important relationship. The watching becomes a high that is valued more than family and friends. Addicts rationalize that they are doing no harm by just watching.

Prostitution

Every now and then a vice squad will close in on an outcall service that has made prostitutes available to customers by phone. Records are seized. A chill goes through the city. Eight to ten thousand people wonder if their names were kept on file. The newspaper accentuates this fear by printing the police comment that the list of patrons included prominent government officials, religious leaders, and businesspeople. Each patron fears that his or her name has surfaced. All rehearse confessions and stories for their bosses and spouses. The public feels sensation and fear, glimpsing for a moment the large network of people who make prostitution a part of their lives.

Prostitution appears in many forms. Some outcall services are so large they have representatives in the major metropolitan areas of the country. Many have toll-free numbers. There are numerous Web sites that can connect a patron with people who will perform sex acts for money. It's as easy as simply naming where you wish to travel, reading the profiles and reviewing the photos, and then making a connection. If you so desire, you can even ask them to bring cocaine or other illegal drugs. And, if you do not have cash, massage and sauna parlors will be happy to charge their services on major credit cards. Many metropolitan hotels are routinely "worked" by young, often beautiful, prostitutes. Businesses hire public relations "consultants." Listening to a CB radio, one quickly becomes aware of vans and pickups driven by women with handles like "Bunny" or "Snuggles." They work the nation's truck stops and rest areas. These forms of the "oldest profession" do not generate public reaction.

Somehow concern is generated only for the streetwalker who works the bars and streets under the tyranny of a pimp. Or the adolescent runaway who ends up being a prostitute just to survive on the streets. Or the young boy who works as a "chicken" in gay cruising areas. The issue of whether prostitution is a victimless crime goes beyond the scope of this book. Our focus of concern is on the addict whose involvement with prostitution is crippling his or her life.

Addicts who use the Twelve Steps will often joke about going to "Johns Anonymous" because of the prevalence of prostitution in sexual addiction and the usage by prostitutes of the word "john" to describe their customers. Addicts like prostitution because it is an immediate fix with few entanglements. Often it is anonymous. Yet the consequences of prostitution are high. The lies are often elaborate. There is risk of disease. There is the possibility of it becoming public knowledge. Yet, the biggest factor for most addicts is the expense. A habit of three to four visits a week is expensive to sustain. One addict, a physician, used up all the equity from the sale of an expensive home in prostitution.

For family men, even more lies are required to explain where the money has gone. When addicts tell about themselves, their stories are frequently punctuated with deep sobs as they tell of the times when they would come home after spending a hundred dollars on a prostitute, only to realize that their children and wives were doing without something they needed. However, as in all addiction, painful realization does not stop compulsive behavior.

Our understanding of prostitutes needs to be expanded. We are aware of women who sell their services because of financial desperation or a drug habit. We also know the impact of sexual and physical abuse from which prostitutes recycle the dramas of their own early family experiences. We know about runaways and pimps. We have even heard of happy hookers. Less aware are we of the woman addict who buries her pain with sexual obsession. Prostitution, even part time, can be a way to get paid for a compulsive sexual need. Prostitutes who fail to understand this part of themselves find it very difficult to stop. Arousal is connected to power and being paid. Not only is prostitution a way to recycle old abuse, but also the humiliation of the john is a real turn-on. We call this eroticized rage. It is often a big part of the reason why prostitutes become "hooked" on this way of life.

Anonymous Sex

Anonymous sex is often seen as simply illicit behavior, but it is really more complex and often brings with it other issues. Joanna could only be orgasmic and passionate with men she did not know. The more dangerous or degrading the sexual activity was, the better it felt. When she was with a loving, decent, and accomplished man, sex was virtually impossible. Like many survivors of sexual abuse, she was sexually "anorexic," or sex avoidant. To be sexual and intimate with a man she liked was too risky. The betrayal of intimacy in her family meant that she could not do it all with one person. Sexual release could only be found with those who were never candidates to be in her "real" life.

Or consider Jim, a Lutheran seminarian. He went to school

full time and worked part time as a youth director in a parish. He was sensitive, intelligent, and committed to his career. He was also driven by his sexual compulsion. His pattern was to frequent at night a well-known park area by a local river that was known as a gay "cruising" area. He would stand by the same tree each time and allow himself to be picked up. His sexual contacts were in the dark with strangers. He always felt humiliated. One time he was severely beaten. He would consistently have unprotected sex.

What prompted Jim to seek help was not a "river" incident. Rather, he was sexual with one of the young men in the parish he served who had visited him at his apartment. He became aware of how vulnerable he was to a charge of sexual exploitation and in his fear sought therapy. Once in therapy, he realized he really had many issues. First, his homosexual orientation would be a problem in his ministry in the church tradition he was in. This constituted a career crisis. And second, his sexual compulsiveness was an obstacle to developing significant relationships. Moreover, he was engaging in high-risk behaviors, such as having unprotected sex with men he did not know. He was leading a secret life that kept him from all he wanted. And he then jeopardized his career by having sex with an underage person.

For gay or lesbian persons who are also sexual addicts, compulsivity simply compounds problems of acceptance and shame. For the sexual addict whose self-image is already marginal, adding the problems of sexual identity intensifies all sexual issues. The gay man who has eight to ten sexual encounters with different partners during a week's time has little chance to develop a real sense of self because of his loneliness and isolation. If those encounters are under degrading or even dangerous circumstances, self-image suffers further.

Anonymous sex is even more complicated for men who consider themselves heterosexual but are compulsive only in homosexual ways. Steve, for example, saw himself as happily married. During a particularly stressful period, he got involved with a man in a rest room in his office building. He repeated the experience a couple of days later. Within a few months, he was a regular in the "hot johns" in his area. In time he expanded into porn shops, meeting men in the movie booths. This lasted for a period of four years.

Two events brought Steve to therapy. The first was that he met his brother walking through the booths at the porn store. He immediately acknowledged to himself that his brother was as troubled as he. Second, while traveling he had sex with a man in a service station rest room while his wife and kids waited in the car. During therapy Steve realized that seeing his brother recalled all those heavily weighted family messages he carried about sexuality and homosexuality. Finally, he had to recognize that his family life was not happy. Comfortable, but not intimate. The service station episode simply underscored that he was lonely in the midst of those he loved. In therapy he had to wrestle with what his bisexuality was about, the emptiness of his marriage, and the fact that he was depressed.

The point in all three of these stories is that anonymous sex is not simple. It usually represents a complex constellation of issues. For Joanna, Jim, and Steve, compulsive, anonymous sex was a short-term solution to life issues that were being avoided.

The Level One Addict

Level One addicts seldom stay with one behavior category. More common would be an addict for whom prostitution, affairs, visits to porn shops, and occasional visits to hot johns form an overall picture of obsession. The accumulated effect is that the addiction can become the center of the addict's life—rooted in a complex malaise of deceit, isolation, and shame.

Many Level One addicts believe they can control their behavior since it is not constant. They experience episodes in which they simply sexually binge. Then they stop for weeks or even months. A salesman, for example, may only use prostitutes when he travels. In town, he perceives his life as "normal." Vows to quit made upon return from his last trip are forgotten with the next. Because of the appearance of "normalcy," he rationalizes that he can handle his behavior and that it has no impact on his life. Yet, he truly has a secret world where damaging consequences subtly overtake him. Normal persons do not carry the secrets and shame he does. He does not stop because he cannot.

The problem for the Level One addicts is that they can rationalize that they are not much different from most folks. While they feel unique in desperateness and obsession, the sexual behavior creates few real social consequences. Yet the addicts pay a personal toll in increasing pain and loneliness. The next level of addiction, however, involves clear violations of cultural norms—and, therefore, greater risk. Also, greater excitement.

Level Two

Level Two addictive behaviors are sufficiently intrusive to warrant stiff legal sanctions. Exhibitionism, voyeurism, indecent phone calls, and indecent liberties all are punished when actively prosecuted. Both prosecutors and the general public, however, view these acts as nuisance offenses. The offenders are seen as pathetic and usually unable to establish effective relationships.[2] Yet there are victims and there are sanctions. The consequences and danger are clearly part of the addictive process. Common to all Level Two obsessions is that someone is victimized.

Exhibitionism

Gene Abel of the New York State Psychiatric Institute reports exhibitionist clients who have exposed themselves two to three hundred times with few or no arrests.[3] There is consensus about the reasons. Fear of reporting, indifference, and cynicism about impact are a few. One of the biggest reasons is that victims seldom get accurate descriptions. The result is that an addict's actions can go unchecked for quite some time. Therefore, what starts as some experimentation can quickly become a flourishing addiction with little interference.

Stereotypically, a flasher is a person who wears a raincoat on sunny days. However, the truth is that exhibitionists are remarkably diverse in their methods, such as

- driving or parking in a car with pants pulled down
- leaving the pants' zipper open and standing in an elevator, on a street, or in a phone booth
- having a "strategic" hole in a pair of jeans or shorts
- wearing swimming trunks without liners
- leaving curtains "inadvertently" ajar in bedroom or bathroom
- ringing a doorbell in a secluded doorway and exposing when it is answered
- walking exposed in shopping malls, campuses, or other open areas
- approaching a building with large windows such as a library or an apartment building and exposing through the window

There are many people who witness an act of exposing who are either unaware of the exhibitionist's intention or dismiss their own judgment as "paranoia." To expose without raising alarm becomes part of the challenge for the exhibitionist. It also limits the consequences of the addiction. The Internet has significantly reduced the risks of exposing and voyeurism. Dedicated Web sites offer the opportunity to post pictures of oneself, one's partner, and couples together. Voyeurs can post nude snapshots of neighbors, relatives, ex-wives, and girlfriends without their consent or knowledge. Cuseeme (see-you-see-me) technology allows people to send live provocative pictures of themselves to others from the safety of their homes. There are those who like the "edge" of exposing this way to people who did not request the photo and are shocked by the image. Yet Net nudism is commonplace on the Internet today.

The method involving the highest risk for the exposer is the use of an automobile. Victims often have sufficient presence of mind to get a license number. Yet driving is a common method. The addict can escape quickly in a car if necessary and can cover more ground in search of women. Exhibitionists who drive while exposing almost invariably report car accidents as one of the consequences of their addiction. They are totally entranced by their approach to their victim and simply do not watch where they are going.

For the exhibitionist whose pattern involves driving, simply entering a car becomes a cue to start the ritual. Scanning streets for potential "scores" becomes almost part of driving. Certain streets and areas become routes that are regularly checked. The addict cannot trust that he will arrive at his intended destination, because driving itself has become a real part of the ritual. Some addicts count making it to work on time a major victory, for once an addict begins cruising, three to six hours may go by before he stops.

The human cost is incredible. Exhibitionists lead double lives. They live with the constant fear that someone who has seen them in their street roles will recognize them in their "other" lives. Worse, they judge themselves by the same standards society uses—as weird, nuisance perverts. That judgment is not accurate, since there is trauma for the victim. Being accosted by an exposer can be very damaging and frightening. Even most exhibitionists carry an image of the face of a person they know they've hurt. Both society and the addict underestimate the danger and the cost of the addiction.

Voyeurism

"Peeping Toms," like flashers, have their stereotypes. The ineffectual bachelor peering into the neighboring apartment via the telescope may seem harmless. For voyeur addicts, however, peeping is usually not their only compulsive behavior. Quite often, they become involved in other addictive behaviors, such as pornography, movies, and strip shows. Moreover, being quite inventive in voyeurism is characteristic. Addicts have many stories about heat vents, mirrors, and cameras. Some of their efforts involve great risk, including peering into house or apartment windows or even hiding in closets.

Over and above the obvious costs, including risk of arrest, most voyeurs agree that one of the biggest losses is time. Watching a window for three or four hours—often under very awkward circumstances—in the hope of glimpsing a minute of nudity is insane even to the addict. Voyeurs report that while waiting, they often struggle with themselves, asking, "Why am I doing this?" They make a commitment to stop waiting by a certain time if nothing happens. Yet the time comes and goes. They sit and continue to wait—until either something does happen or it is obvious that nothing will. Each episode is followed by depression and pain. The loss of time and energy, the deep embarrassment about being a voyeur, and the self-hatred at being unable to control oneself combine to keep an addict absolutely isolated. There is one simple way to alleviate the pain temporarily. Do it again.

As with most addicts, the voyeur is sustained by excitement. He waits in a trancelike state, with energies focused in the waiting. Totally absorbed, the addict loses all contact with reality, save for the focus of the addiction. Cares, worries, deadlines, and responsibilities are for a blessed moment suspended. The mood-altering qualities of the experience are enhanced by the intrusive, the stolen, the illicit parts of the behavior. Objectively, the voyeur could go to the local topless bar and see more with less risk and discomfort. He could have sex with someone who wants to have sex with him. Or he could pay for sex. Or he could use the Internet to subscribe to one of the many Web sites that use Minicams in a house where young women live. But it just doesn't offer the same thrill or risk factor as the other behaviors. The real problem is an essential distortion of courtship. For children, to play "I'll show you mine, you show me yours" is a normal part of growing up. To look and be looked at are normal parts of adult courtship. To show "yours" to people who do not wish to see it or to watch someone who doesn't want to be observed means that the person has eroticized a part of courtship that leaves other aspects of intimacy and sexuality underdeveloped. It is about how the person was damaged while growing up.

The excitement of illicit victimization is rooted in the addicts' anger about that hurt. Breaking the rules is a way to retaliate for hurts, real and imagined. The anger stems from a set of beliefs, family messages, and self-judgments the addicts use to interpret the world. Most addicts do not connect their behavior with anger. The excitement and arousal of the trance block the feelings, along with the rest of the pain.

The greater the anger and pain, the more excitement is required to block it. This dynamic is the key to understanding how escalation occurs within the addictive process. If the current behavior within the addictive cycle is no longer supplying the excitement necessary to block the pain, something with greater risk is attempted. A good example is the addict who is a combination voyeur-exhibitionist.

The Voyeur-Exhibitionist

Voyeurism and exhibitionism often go together. The connecting link is masturbation. For the voyeur, masturbating while watching is another way of enhancing the excitement.

The addict finds a position in which he can watch attractive women walk by, but in which he cannot be seen. This is usually a car, a first-floor rest room, office, or bedroom, or even a portable satellite toilet like those commonly found at beaches, parks, and rest areas. The thrill is in ejaculating within a few feet of a woman without her knowledge. Masturbating in front of her is but a fragile step away.

Pete is an addict who took that step. His sexual history from the seventh grade on was characterized by compulsive masturbation and involvement with many girls or women at the same time. He met a woman, Angie, with whom he fell in love in his junior year of college. They were married shortly after his graduation.

Pete landed a job as a salesman for a large grain firm. Because of his potential as a businessman, he was given a huge territory with very little guidance as to how to manage it. Accountability was high, but only on a semiannual basis. The result was that Pete had a lot of unstructured time and very little support. He was totally overwhelmed.

Although he had only been married a little while, he was already feeling restless. His sexual relationship with Angie was excellent, yet he missed his "woman-chasing." Late one night, he went for a walk. Noting an open window, he found himself watching a neighborhood teenager undress. It was the greatest sexual arousal he could remember. This event initiated a year of intense voyeurism all over the city.

Pete had an extraordinary gift of gab, and people trusted him. Nonetheless, his charm could not cover his neglect of his job. His boss transferred him to a less demanding territory, but equally unstructured. Pete felt demoralized. He saw himself as a procrastinator. He also blamed his peeping, which was taking a lot of his energy. He was committed to proving himself in his job, but repeated efforts to stop his voyeurism failed.

Pete's sexual demands on his wife were increasing and becoming more insensitive. Angie was starting to complain about being pestered. Angie and Pete also had a baby, so that Angie's energy was absorbed in child care. Pete felt abandoned at a time when he was now the sole financial support of the family.

One summer night, Pete had parked near a college campus. He was watching the windows of the women's dorm. He also enjoyed watching and listening as the young women walked past his car. He started masturbating in the car. It was exhilarating. He soon started driving around at night masturbating and exposing himself. In a short time he tried this activity in the daytime. To his surprise, some would watch and some would avert their eyes. Nothing else happened.

Within a few weeks, Pete's life was almost totally involved in exposing himself. He would go to work only if there were mandatory meetings he had to attend. Otherwise, he would end up cruising in his car. He began to know the city in a different way—the rhythm of the city in terms of when and where women would be: colleges in the morning, shopping malls at noon, parks and schools in the afternoon. Sometimes he would engage in voyeurism at night.

Usually when he came home, he was exhausted. Sometimes he would go to bed without supper. Angie thought he was overworking. The reality was that his trance-like search coupled with masturbating for hours left him drained.

Like all addicts, Pete became entangled in a complex web—lies and deceits with his boss and with his wife. He had to explain his absences and failure to perform. What was worse was that he had broken his own rule and was becoming involved with a secretary at work. He also visited his first prostitute. He was woman-chasing again.

There were times at the end of an all-day binge when he felt his life was out of control. He would break down sobbing over his steering wheel. He vowed to stop each time. But he would resume, maybe even that night. He often thought of himself as being like a heroin addict.

One spring day he had the peak exhibitionist experience. A young woman had put her head in the window of the car, talked to him, and watched him masturbate to ejaculation. He was still in that transitory mood of elation and peacefulness as he pulled into the driveway. There a squad car was waiting. Angie was on the back steps holding the baby, looking absolutely terrified. The image was burned on his soul, for in one moment the consequences of his addiction were placed in sharp relief against everything he cherished and loved.

Pete got help because of thoughtful police intervention, but not before he lost his job, which happened a few days later. His termination was not related to his arrest, but was obviously connected to his addiction. Usually a full-blown addiction occurs over a long period of time, but Pete's story illustrates how the sexual addiction can destroy a person in less than two years. The escalation of the addiction matches the increasing pain, isolation, and shame. The voyeur-exhibitionist combination is a potent illustration. Another set of Level Two behaviors that share the same process is usually called "indecent" by society.

Indecent Calls and Liberties

Indecent phone calls occur when the addict calls a woman in order to make suggestive statements, to ask intrusive or embarrassing sexual questions, or to assault her verbally. Or consider the woman who reveals inappropriate things about herself to someone she does not know. Compared with the voyeur-exhibitionist, the difference is that victimization occurs visually with one and orally with the other. Masturbation can serve as an important link here as well. Addicts may start by masturbating while talking on the phone to someone who is not aware of it. Soon, however, efforts to be more explicit about the sexual intrusion can follow.

Indecent liberties are inappropriate touches, sometimes referred to as minirapes. Here, too, addicts follow a path of escalating addiction. In the press of a crowded subway or shopping mall, the brush of a hand against a thigh or breast can be regarded as accidental. In the rush, it is hard not to bump into someone. Addicts tell stories about what they would do to "have accidents" in the company of their spouses or children. Loved ones become a cover—the incongruity of which adds to the addicts' shame. All the ingredients are present: the stolen, the illicit, the exciting.

Escalation with indecent liberties takes a significant departure. Touching others with their knowledge but without their permission is the next step. For a woman to know clearly that she has been fondled against her will creates a level of intrusion that is truly frightening. Society's response to the sexual abuse is that a nuisance has been transformed into a punishable personal violation. The addict knows that fact. To be compulsive to that degree in spite of the obvious consequences is to propel the addict into Level Three sexual behavior.

Level Three

The common element of Level Three behavior is that some of our most significant boundaries are violated. Rape, incest, and child molesting are basic transgressions of laws designed to protect the vulnerable. There is little compassion or understanding for someone compulsive at this level. Yet, addiction exists here too. Whether or not there *should* be compassion or understanding is another issue. That addiction exists here is a fact.

Child Molesting and Incest

The addict who focuses on children usually has suffered some interruption in his or her own development while growing up. There is a part of the addict that is not any older than the victim. Actual behavior may span all three levels of addiction, including compulsive masturbation with child pornography, child prostitution, voyeuristic and exposing behavior with children, and molestation. There are child molesters who are compulsive with adults as well. In those situations, the addict has a preference—either child before adult, or adult before child. Further complicating factors reside in the sexual identity of the addict, that is, man or woman, homosexual or heterosexual.

The sexual abuse of children has a long history far beyond the scope of this book. As our awareness grows of its extent, the more we know of its damage. Abuse is a major factor in the transmission of sexual compulsivity from one generation to the next. Nowhere is this more evident than in the family where incest takes place.

What a child learns from a parent is how to have a relationship. When a parent is sexual with a child, the child concludes at a fundamental level that in order to have a relationship, one has to be sexual. Thus, all relationships become sexualized. Fathers and mothers are naturally attracted to their children. One of the gifts of parenthood is not to act on those feelings. Those who argue for the right of children to be sexual with their parents miss the developmental point.

Vern was intensely active sexually with his two daughters for an eight-year period. The fact did not come out until his family was brought in during his treatment for alcoholism. He knew his behavior was wrong and had struggled repeatedly to stop. As part of his therapy, Vern had to confront the fact that he had been sexually abused by both his mother and father. When talking with his dad, who was still alive, he discovered that the abuse transcended four generations. His father, too, had been abused. Vern also had to acknowledge that his sexual addiction extended to pornography, many affairs, and extensive involvement with prostitutes.

A situation similar to incest exists for professionals such as physicians or therapists, whose patients are like children in their vulnerability. For the professional to be sexual with them is also to betray a trust. The sexual addict who exploits professional client relationships is in reality committing a type of incest.

Remember, however, behavior by itself does not make an addict. Further, to have feelings of attraction for a child (or a client) does not constitute addiction. Even to act on those feelings, as damaging as that would be, does not make an addict. Addicts are people who cannot stop their behavior, which is crippling them and those around them.

Rape and Violence

Violent fantasies are common in human beings. These fantasies reflect cultural attitudes that see force and violence as an inevitable part of human sexuality. Feminists have long been outspoken critics of abusive norms in our "sick society." Their criticisms have a solid empirical basis. Neil Malamuth, a psychologist from the University of Manitoba, writes:

> Research we and other investigators have conducted strongly supports the feminist viewpoint. It has been found that within the normal population many men have the type of physiological, attitudinal, and behavioral tendencies paralleling those of rapists. Moreover, the belief system of both males and females clearly shows a pattern that condones the use of force in sexual relationships.[4]

Clearly, rape and violence are the tips of a large cultural iceberg.

If many people have the potential for violence, what is it that brings some to the point of rape? Some argue that rape stems from a fundamental lawlessness. One of the very best surveys of the literature on this subject is *Sex, Crime, and the Law* by Donald MacNamara and Edward Sagarin, stating:

> Most arrests are of males of low social-economic status, and the fact that such a high percentage of the rapists had also been arrested for property crimes would strongly suggest a ghetto or poverty background and a general orientation of disrespect for the law. More important, they are in the main not people who are

psychopathically involved as oversexualized beings or persons with uncontrollable sexual impulses. With few exceptions, they do not seem to be career rapists, or even "career sex criminals," although they might be seen as career criminals.[5]

While MacNamara and Sagarin describe an important perspective on the overall issue of rape, another way to view rape is to see it as part of a general pattern of compulsivity. Rape can be the most extreme expression of escalation in the sexual addiction. However, not all rapists are addicts, but some addicts are rapists. A good example is the case of George. George was an appliance repairman. He was extremely skillful at figuring out how to make things work again. He took pride in that. He was also proud of his wife, son, and three daughters. The secret in the family was George's alcoholism, which everyone shielded from the outside world. The family attributed its problems to his drinking. For the outside world, his craftsmanship and his dependability were well recognized. He was Catholic and served several terms as parish trustee.

George led another life as well—the life of a sexual addict in the advanced stages. About two years before he was married, George had been arrested for exhibitionism. Now at the age of forty-three, he had been arrested again. His secret life was revealed and he was forced into treatment. His therapist required that George complete alcoholism treatment first. Then George started on treatment for his sexual addiction.

George's list of sexual compulsivity was lengthy. Compulsive masturbation, usually with pornography, voyeurism, and exhibitionism were weekly and sometimes daily events. He had many affairs, including one with a customer that lasted four years. One of his "secrets" involved his being so trustworthy that his customers would leave him alone in the house to do repair work. He liked to explore dresser drawers and finger underclothing, panties, and bras. Prostitution was a major part of his lifestyle. At one point, he had to obtain a secret loan for $2,700 to cover withdrawals he had made to pay for prostitutes. In the year before his arrest, George had also raped six women at knifepoint. He had physically molested seven others.

George's story is not atypical. Compulsive rapists report the presence of many Level One and Two behaviors as part of their paths. This does not mean that sexual addiction leads inexorably to being a rapist. It does mean that to see prostitution, pornography, exhibitionism, and voyeurism as mere nuisances is to misunderstand the nature of sexual addiction. Some addicts commit rape as part of their overall compulsivity.

Another example is the story of Bill, who was referred by a criminal justice diversion project for his exhibitionism. Shortly after beginning therapy he was referred to a hospital inpatient program for his alcoholism. After treatment, he rejoined his therapy group for dealing with his sexual addiction. He initially maintained that his exhibitionism was limited to driving around masturbating in his car. He eventually admitted to a twelve-year history of exhibitionism. In addition, he told of numerous affairs, in one of which he fathered a child. Prostitution was also a significant part of his history. With the group's assistance he was able to calculate that he had spent in excess of thirty thousand dollars on prostitutes within a three-year period. Given that he had a limited income, his prostitution habit alone was a severe strain on his family.

Beginning with Bill's treatment for his alcoholism, his wife and four children became involved in therapy. Bill began to get reacquainted with his children. His wife continued a cold and distant hostility. Very seldom would she comment or become involved. She saw it clearly as his problem and believed that "things would change if he did." It was not until Bill revealed that he was also a rapist that things changed in the family. The pain was so great for Ginger, his wife, that she, too, came into therapy.

For a month, it was doubtful if the family would stay together. With serious effort by all involved, relationships improved. After seventeen months in the program, the marriage was rewarding for both; Bill was staying straight in all of his addictions and had recently been made a supervisor in his company. Keys to the recovery were honesty, recognition of all the levels of addiction, and total family involvement. As an indication of how essential these elements are, the following is an edited excerpt from Bill's account of what he had done:

> I think of all the Saturday and Sunday mornings that I would sneak off, sometimes in the afternoon or evenings. But the sneakiest way was before anybody got up. That way I did not have to explain where I was going—only the lie as to where I had been when I got back home. "Where have you been all morning or all day?" Some of the lies were, "Oh, I was over to a friend's house," sometimes even making up a friend. Or the countless times that I had car trouble and how hard and long it was to fix. If asked about the friend, it was somebody from work: "You would not know him, anyway you never met him." [He gives an example of a mud slide after a hard rain and helping an imaginary friend fix a wall that caved in.] Sometimes I got mad because she asked where I was. I said, "None of your business."
>
> There were countless times where I came to work late, left early, or did not show up at all. I told my boss I was sick or something happened at home. Spending endless

hours driving around. I would leave the house on the spur of the moment with a lie to get in my car and go.

I could be driving down the street with good intentions. Just a thought or the sight of a pretty girl would get me going. I would tell myself it is not going to happen, but did not have any control to stop it. Completely powerless, a feeling of being taken over by a strong emotionally uncontrollable power that I did not understand. Afterwards, I would feel so ashamed of what I had done and then starting right in over again, maybe even staying out all night or even looking for a prostitute.

Sometimes after the prostitute and driving home thinking about the prostitute, it would start in all over again; just the thought. I would get home and wonder why I had done it. Then not knowing where I was at, what I had been doing. Or being caught by someone I knew or somebody else knew, like the time my daughter's friend saw my picture at the police department. Plus, explaining where my money went when I had put it in the gas tank and all the nicks in the car.

I would sometimes wonder what the girl or woman thought or the remark they would make if they saw me, "Goddamn creep, queen, sex maniac, etc." You can well imagine how apart I was from my family because of the guilty feeling; shamefulness for time away from home; sad because of all of it. Angry at myself for not doing anything about it or being able to control it. Why am I this way, why me? How can a person live that way for ten to twelve years and face themselves? Knowing what you are, the deep down truth crawling around in the back of your mind and the pit of your stomach. Everybody looks at you and you're not able to look at them. Dear God help me.

To rape out of anger, passion, or lawlessness—as terrible as that is—does not constitute an addiction. There are some sexual addicts, however, for whom rape is part of a larger pattern. Once past our rage for what has been done, we can see rape as the most tragic extension of the addict's world.

COROLLARIES OF THE LEVELS OF ADDICTION

The levels of addiction are arbitrary concepts. They serve, however, to show the wide range of behavior included in sexual addiction. While our discussion did not extend to every possible form of the addiction (e.g., bestiality, sado-masochism, and fetishism were omitted), the levels provide a basic strategy for understanding any sexually compulsive behavior. Most important, the levels make explicit the pattern created by the relationship between behaviors. See the chart Levels of Addiction, which follows on pages 66 and 67.

Many concepts are limited when applied to real life. The levels are no different. The incestuous father who combines bestiality with his dog with the sexual abuse of his daughters, the exhibitionist who spends time with his family in the nudist camp, the physician voyeur who does routine physicals as part of his practice—all are situations difficult to assess within the three levels. The value of the levels of addiction remains in their ability to underline the patterns of compulsive sexuality.

Just as the levels serve as a basic premise about the extent of addiction, there are five corollaries, listed here, that are critical to understanding the addiction. Each of the five must be recognized if the levels of addiction are to be useful tools in the assessment of any individual's addiction.

LEVEL OF ADDICTION	BEHAVIOR	CULTURAL STANDARDS
Level One	Masturbation, compulsive relationships, pornography, prostitution, and anonymous sex	Depending on behavior, activities are seen as acceptable or tolerable. Some specific behaviors such as prostitution and homosexuality are sources of controversy.
Level Two	Exhibitionism, voyeurism, indecent phone calls, and indecent liberties	None of these behaviors is acceptable.
Level Three	Child molestation, incest, and rape	Each behavior represents a profound violation of cultural boundaries.

Figure 2.1

ADDICTION

LEGAL CONSEQUENCES/ RISKS	VICTIM	PUBLIC OPINION OF ADDICTION
Sanctions against those behaviors, when illegal, are ineffectively and randomly enforced. Low priority for enforcement officials generates minimal risk for addict.	These behaviors are perceived as victimless crimes. However, victimization and exploitation are often components.	Public attitudes are characterized by ambivalence or dislike. For some behaviors such as prostitution there is a competing negative hero image of glamorous decadence.
Behaviors are regarded as nuisance offenses. Risk is involved since offenders, when observed, are actively prosecuted.	There is always a victim.	Addict is perceived as pathetic and sick but harmless. Often these behaviors are the objects of jokes that dismiss the pain of the addict.
Extreme legal consequences create high-risk situations for the addict.	There is always a victim.	Public becomes outraged. Perpetrators are seen by many as subhuman and beyond help.

Corollary One: The sexual addiction of each level is painful.

The pain at each level is very real. The problem is that the public, addicts, and others dismiss the pain, but for different reasons at different levels. A macho society would perceive an unending string of lovers and prostitutes as simply having a good time. Level One behavior may even be envied or, at the minimum, regarded as normal but not as painful. Similarly, the nuisance offenders of Level Two are dismissed as pathetic and harmless or as the object of jokes (e.g., "flasher" jokes), but not as haunted, wounded, or broken people. Level Three behavior engenders such immediate rage that rapists, molesters, and incestuous fathers justifiably receive no quarter. There is much compassion for the victim, but no sense of the desperation of the addict.

Some time ago there was an episode of the TV show *Police Woman* that illustrated the stereotypic ways in which the pain of the addiction is dismissed. The plot of the story was about the chase and capture of two rapists. The rapists were brothers who were portrayed as cruel, vicious low-life types who, by any viewer's standards, would deserve the very worst.

In the midst of the chase, a subplot emerged designed for comic relief. Into the station walked a man who had been pinching women on elevators and could not stop. In desperation, he turned himself in. The contrast was intended to be comical. However, addicts who have thought of turning themselves in as a way out of their predicament had to find the episode disconcerting. Addicts can only guess at how they will be accepted by authorities.

Pathos, rage, and idealization of the male sexual role—all obscure the addict's pain. Without a sense of the addict's loneliness, shame, and despair, none of the levels of sexual compulsiveness can be appreciated as an addiction.

Corollary Two: Deviant behavior does not necessarily indicate the presence of addiction.

Throughout this chapter, a constant theme has been that a pattern is necessary for addiction to exist. Rape and incest, for example, are tragic, but they are not necessarily the result of addiction. Deviancy, however, does involve risk. Risk does seem to be one of the prime ingredients to the mood-altering addictive process. To violate cultural and legal norms can enhance the sexual excitement. Risk, which is involved in the violation, is central to the escalation process so often described by addicts. Therefore, the presence of deviant behavior warrants exploring the possibility of sexual addiction.

Corollary Three: All three levels of addiction transcend personality, gender, and socioeconomic status.

At this time, it is difficult to make descriptive statements about sexual addicts with empirical certainty. We do not know, for example, how many addicts there are in general, let alone how many addicts within specific levels. There is no survey technique that can guarantee total candor about sexual behavior across the levels. Nor has there been, heretofore, an integrating concept—such as addiction—that makes connections within patterns of behavior for researchers to use. Finally, studies of sexual compulsiveness often are done within the criminal justice system. Obviously, total honesty brings risk in that situation. The stories of members of Twelve Step groups and the case histories of those who have been forced into treatment or who have sought help voluntarily are our best sources to date. Their experiences suggest that the addiction has few limits, transcending personality, gender, and socioeconomic status.

Personality studies of people with sexually compulsive behavior have had only limited success in specifying personality
characteristics.[6] Psychological test data, clinical observation,
and case studies usually indicate that there is no outstanding
similarity in personality factors. Convincing arguments are
difficult to find for any kind of general personality type, even
within a specific category of compulsivity. In addition, researchers often have only small groups to study, do not look at
overall sexual patterns, and ignore the presence of multiple
addictions. Research is further complicated by the delusional
thought processes of addicts, who, in fact, are not aware of the
extent of their problems. A long time elapses before recovering
addicts have clarity, let alone before they are able and willing
to describe their past situations to others.

Like alcoholism, the sexual addiction may include many
variations of personality and even personality disorders. As
suggested in chapter 1, concurrent emotional illness is often
part of the addict's world. The levels of addiction highlight
the fact that we can no longer generalize about the shy flasher,
the hard-core rapist, the sex-starved john, or the socially inept
incestuous parent. Sexual addiction can flourish in the most
competent, attractive, and charming people as well as in the
most retiring, repulsive, and ill.

Nor can we assume that sexual addiction is a lower-class
phenomenon. The case examples used in the writing of this
book represent a broad spectrum of class, profession, and educational experience. Within the public media, there is a constant parade of key public figures who have been exposed for
their sexual compulsiveness:

- A high-ranking federal official was arrested for sexual
  activities in a Washington, D.C., bookstore.
- A state supreme court judge, nationally recognized for

his legal scholarship, was exposed by a television news team for his activities with teenage homosexual prostitutes.

- One of the aerospace engineers who helped design the space shuttle was cited for incest with his children.

- The president and chief executive officer of one of the largest family-owned manufacturing companies was exposed as the central figure in a large child pornography network.

- A minister and high-ranking official of a large Protestant denomination was arrested for exhibitionism.

The sensationalism that surrounds these cases obscures the fact that the consequences of sexual addiction may fall harder on addicts with less money and access to legal assistance. Contrast the sexual activities of a dot.com billionaire with a working man who has only enough money to pick up street "hookers." The latter is clearly less protected. Professionals are beginning to wonder if the extent of sexual compulsiveness among those with more resources has been underestimated. For example, professionals are now reporting to the National Center on Child Abuse and Neglect (NCCAN) an increasing number of cases of sexual abuse among middle- and upper-income families.

The levels of addiction also provide a more complete perspective on sexual addiction for women. Men are clearly perceived as capable of being obsessive about sex. Because of the sexual exploitation of women, the image of women alleviating their pain through sexual obsession is more rare. Yet our media is filled with examples like Mrs. Robinson in *The Graduate*, Theresa in *Looking for Mr. Goodbar*, or the desperate women in *American Gigolo*. Sexual compulsiveness exists for women on each level of the addiction. The woman who repeatedly uses objects to masturbate to the point of injury, the woman "flasher" who hikes her dress and opens the car door to expose herself to passing men, and the woman who has been sexual with four out of her six children—all can share a common addictive process.

There are special problems for women addicts. There are the risks of violence and pregnancy. There is the double standard for the sexual behavior of women. There are the conflicting messages of cultural norms. A woman in a bikini or a low-cut gown is idolized and a stripper is degraded. Men addicts ask, "Why, when a man looks at a woman in a window, he is a voyeur, and when a woman looks at a man in a window, he is an exhibitionist?" Setting aside the rage for women implicit in the question, it does raise the problem of public attitudes toward women.

Consider the woman who exposes herself in public. The reactions will probably be less punitive than for a man. Yet, given the cultural role of women as guardians of sexual morality, the shame is greater. Similar dynamics exist for women who have multiple affairs or are sexual with children. Their recovery is made harder because of the messages incorporated in their belief systems about how a woman "should" be. Even to admit there is a sexual problem is more difficult. To reject the reality of sexual addiction for women is to perpetuate the sexism that has prevented women with other addictions from receiving help in the past.

Corollary Four: Sexual behaviors within and between levels reinforce one another.

Within the levels of behaviors, the addict will shift from one behavior to another depending on availability, risk, and situation. The salesman feels safer entering a massage parlor or bookstore on the road than at home. Masturbating while looking at pornography can suffice when the addict has failed to make the evening pickup at the local bars. The addict who makes indecent phone calls and is worried about arrest can now call a phone service. One-half hour of explicit sexual conversation with a young woman while masturbating can be charged to his credit card.

An example of how behavior can shift within the addictive cycle was shared by a woman who worked in a massage parlor. She reported that recently there had been a rape of one of the masseuses in the place she worked. When she went to the police station to examine mug shots of sex offenders, she was stunned to discover that she was able to recognize a large number of the pictures—they were her clients. It was shortly thereafter that she entered therapy.

Corollary Five: Sexual behavior in each level is connected with behaviors due to other kinds of addiction.

The pattern of sexual behavior is not complete unless the reinforcement of other compulsive behaviors is counted. Overeating, working, and drinking or abusing drugs are integral to the addict's pattern. This is true, for example, when

- working until exhausted justifies sexual compulsiveness as "deserved"
- drinking and cruising are mutually intoxicating
- binge eating routinely follows a visit to a porn shop
- gambling and prostitution are an irresistible combination
- cocaine and sex are only used together

Just as the sexual behaviors on each level reinforce each other, other addictions play an important role in conjunction with each other. The interaction between addictions may be at just one level. Consider the incestuous father who is also an alcoholic. His compulsive masturbation, use of pornography, or use of prostitutes did not have to involve drinking. Yet every time he was sexual with his daughter he was also drunk. The two addictions come together at Level Three, but not Level One. Addicts must discern the total pattern in order to understand their powerlessness and unmanageability.

ADDICTION AS A SYSTEM

Traditionally, sexual compulsiveness has been described in a linear fashion. Behavior was divided into types and categories, with each having its own origin. Exhibitionists were one way, incestuous fathers were another, and the unfaithful spouse yet another. Undoubtedly each behavior has unique characteristics. The difficulty in gathering data plus the shame and denial system of the addict perpetuate the idea that each individual category is unique. However, for true addicts there is a common link in sexual obsession.

The addiction is truly a system where behavior is interdependent. There are constantly shifting patterns that weave together the various levels of sexually compulsive behavior and that may include other addictions and emotional disorders. The system operates on a repetitive rhythm. The driving force for each cycle comes from a faulty belief system translated through delusional thought patterns. In general, systems are self-perpetuating, and the sexual addiction as a system is just that. The completion of each cycle confirms that belief system and the impaired thinking. Out of the validation of the beliefs a new and stronger cycle is born. The behavior, then, becomes intensified within Level One, and sometimes extends to Levels Two and Three.

In recent years, cybersex has become a large factor in sex addiction. There is literally nothing described in this chapter that cannot be facilitated by the Internet. It is vital to understand the role of the computer as an accelerator of addictive behavior. This is the focus of the next chapter.

CHAPTER 3

Cybersex and Addictive Behavior

◩ ◩ ◩

> Robert Glass . . . pleaded guilty Thursday to strangling a
> woman during sex after they met in an online chatroom in
> 1996.
>
> —*Charlotte Observer*, January 2000

> A mayoral candidate who abruptly dropped out of the race
> last month had been arrested a day earlier on charges of solic-
> iting sex on the Internet.
>
> —*Arizona Republic*, February 2000

> A French woman who was wooed on the Internet, then trav-
> eled to meet her suitor, was found dead in an apparent suicide
> after the man used her for sex and kicked her out, police said.
>
> —Associated Press, 2000

It was 2:00 A.M. John sat at his desk staring at the screen of his
computer. His pain was indescribable. He had been surfing the
Net, going from one pornographic Web site to another. His
wife, Susan, had gone to bed at about 9:30 P.M. He started
surfing the Net at 10:00 P.M., However, he did not start masturbating until 11:00 P.M., after he was sure his wife was soundly
asleep. He hated what he was doing, but once he entered
the cyberworld of "anything goes," all his sexual longings

exploded. It was beyond pleasure. He never knew how much desire he was capable of until he discovered the secret world of cybersex. Every curiosity, fantasy, and perverse thought could be explored. At times he would just ache when circumstances prevented his almost daily sessions at the computer.

This particular evening, his views regarding cybersex changed abruptly when he entered a voyeur Web site where people post nude photos of their spouses or of themselves. As he anxiously flipped through the archives, John was stunned to see a photo posted of someone he recognized. It was of his daughter-in-law, Connie, the mother of his two young grand-children. There she was with her breasts fully exposed as she smiled at the camera demurely. She was provocatively remov-ing her jeans, and the caption written by his own son, James, teased the viewer: "Tell us that you like what you see, and maybe I can get her to do more."

In every life there are moments of extraordinary clarity. In one striking moment, John had hit just such a nexus. Clearly John's son, James, was on the same path that he was. John knew firsthand what it was like to constantly pressure your spouse to do things you would both regret later. Once John had entered into the trancelike world of cybersex, it became extremely im-portant to have a cooperating spouse. In cyberspace, a different set of rules prevailed in which it was arousing to have others lust after your spouse. Posting pictures of her made her inter-esting again. John realized that his son and daughter-in-law were participating in an activity that could have extraordinary negative consequences. John wondered why they didn't bother to blur Connie's face so she could remain anonymous. But in re-ality, he knew this would not cover the deeper issues. Still, John was stunned at his son's behavior since James was a prominent pediatrician and his practice depended on the appearance of wholesomeness. James and Connie would be ostracized from their church in an instant if found out. Further, in their very conservative denomination, their actions would disrupt the very fabric of their lives. Nothing had ever given John any indication that his son shared his sexual obsession. He had often admired his son for not having "a monkey on his back." Now he knew his son's secret. And he could only guess at the rest.

Things were getting complicated fast. His initial feelings of arousal were replaced with fear. John's first impulse was to immediately wake up his wife and show her the photo of Connie. But then he worried about tarnishing his own reputation. He knew he could never really explain how he stumbled upon that photo on the Internet. After all, he prided himself as being a hard-working CEO whose integrity was beyond question. Further, he couldn't trust his ability to maintain the lie with her. This incident would open up a whole lot of inquiries. After all, both John and his wife had dealt with some painful sexual issues in the past. This discovery of Connie's photo had the potential to jeopardize John's secret world on the Internet, his one refuge from all the pressure of daily life. John knew what he had to do. Nothing. The costs were simply too high.

By now, John was spending about thirty hours a week having cybersex. He was squeezing cybersex into his day whenever he had an opportunity to be on the computer unobserved. John's company was going public, and employees, investors, and his family had a lot riding on this one important transaction. On the crucial day the company went public, John spent six hours in his office, with the door locked, having cybersex. Everyone thought he was diligently preparing for his press conferences. Now he can barely remember what he said and how he even got through the press conferences that followed.

John was no stranger to infidelity. The Internet now provided more opportunities for betrayal. He was exchanging romantic e-mails with two women, both of whom were married. John deliberately chose married women to become involved with because they had too much to lose to breach the secret of their liaison. John thought his deliberate actions were both clever and predatory. His dealings with the new human resources director were another story. John had spent many hours working closely with her. She confessed two weeks ago how much she loved him and how trapped she felt in her crumbling marriage. They had not yet had sex because they both agreed their actions could destroy John's company. But they fondled each other while they had this intimate discussion. John wondered if James had experienced similar devastating sexual encounters.

Troubled finances were another issue. In truth, John was precariously close to bankruptcy. He had bought this company while it was in serious trouble, mainly to keep its owner quiet—a woman with whom he had been having an affair. The company continued to lose huge sums of money, and John covered it with his own retirement funds. This, in turn, had cost him additional income taxes. He had also overinvested in his company and was manipulating the accounting books to keep nervous bankers satisfied. He had not shared any of this financial information with his wife. He knew that if she had access to their personal and business finances, she would certainly discover the secret life that John was living. John soon discovered that once you lie in one area, it becomes easier to lie in others. For a man whose reputation was built on honesty, this seemed crazy.

As he had been thinking about all this, he realized that he had spent the last thirty minutes gazing at the breasts of his daughter-in-law on the computer screen. "I must be insane," he thought. In fact, if sanity is the ability to face reality, he was insane.

THE CYBERSEX REVOLUTION

How does cybersex get to be such a problem for people? Anonymity is a huge factor. People can be anyone they want on the Internet. They forgo the risk of being seen while visiting a porn shop or local massage parlor. They can download all the pornography they can handle, in their own home, for free. They can schedule prostitutes online, look at their prostitutes' photos and bios, and even talk with them from their own home or office. The risk of being discovered is lowered. They can access almost any type of sexual behavior, even if they have low-level computer skills. If it is sexual, it can be found somewhere on the Net. All three levels of sexually addictive behavior (Level One: behaviors that are regarded as normal, acceptable, or tolerable; Level Two: behaviors that are clearly victimizing and for which legal sanctions are enforced; and Level Three: behaviors that have grave consequences for the victims and legal consequences for the addicts) can be intensified by the Internet. Many of the risks have simply been removed.

Denial is also a factor. Compulsive cybersex users rely on impaired thinking—the type of delusions sex addicts have always had. Addicts start telling themselves that cybersex is not real because it is only "virtual." Often they rationalize that having cybersex is similar to playing a virtual reality computer game. They might rationalize by saying, "I am not really being unfaithful because the person is not real." So the logic goes that no one is hurt—including themselves. As a result, addicts view cybersex use as having no consequences. With this impaired thinking, addicts believe that they can stop whenever they want.

Cybersex reality is different than fantasy. It can have all the hallmarks of addiction. People start spending a lot of time—

time they can ill afford—on the Internet. Soon they begin to regret it. The Internet has an extraordinary capacity to induce a trancelike state. People will spend hours on the Internet in which they lose track of time—and reality. Sexual obsession and the processes of preoccupation and ritualization are engaged. Before cybersex, sex addicts told stories about how they would repeatedly watch a particular pornographic video or drive up and down specific streets as part of their obsession. Preoccupation and ritualization distort judgment so much that being self-destructive somehow makes sense. In the addictive system, preoccupation and ritualization make sexual compulsion inevitable (see figure 1.1 on page 26). For the cybersex addict, even the sound of the modem starting becomes sexualized and ritualistic. The addicts' computer trance bypasses logic, and they find themselves doing things they never imagined. Computers provided new technology for our oldest obsessions.

Consider the case of Dorie, a professional woman with several graduate degrees. She was smart and successful, with a very important leadership role in a large hospital system. She was also married and the mother of two children. Behind her professional exterior, she also was a romance junkie constantly falling in love. She knew she had a problem. An example of her obsession was when she became preoccupied with a doctor at work. She imagined herself in an intense affair with him for nine months. Her obsession caused her to shift her work assignments to be with him, work side-by-side with him as often as possible, think about him constantly, and become very aroused just being in his presence. In reality, while all this was going on, the doctor had no idea she felt that way about him. The affair was totally in her mind.

Disgusted and frustrated by the reality of the situation, she turned to the Internet for comfort. Chat-room and e-mail romances blossomed for Dorie. Since travel was a requirement of her work, she started setting up in-person encounters with her e-mail acquaintances. She finally discovered a man she felt was destined to be her partner for life. She decided to surprise him by flying to see him. She told her family she was going to a meeting in a city in Canada, where this man lived. She showed up on his doorstep at 10:00 P.M. unannounced on a cold winter's night. Although surprised and startled to see her, he invited her in. Within minutes they were having sex. After sex, his attitude suddenly changed. He abruptly asked her to leave. She found herself out on the street in the dark, in a neighborhood far from a phone or taxi. How far she had fallen penetrated her as much as the subzero temperatures. She was lost and didn't know where to turn. How could he treat her like this? She never imagined he'd be like this. She thought she knew him. As she stood out in the street, she heard a car approaching. She looked over her shoulder to see a car pull into his driveway. A woman with several children got out. As they approached the house, she knew. That was his family. Reality sank in.

Dorie is not alone. Stanford researcher Al Cooper found that of the most extreme cybersex users, 40 percent are women. The anonymity of the Net allows women to ignore the normal inhibitions that keep them safe. In fact, many women do not just walk away like Dorie. They put themselves in high-risk situations with men they do not know, resulting in beatings and even murder. In one Colorado case, a woman became involved with a man on the Internet who kidnapped her for six weeks and then murdered her. Another woman traveled all the way from Paris to meet her lover. After having sex with her, he kicked her out and she committed suicide in the frigid winter snow. Notice that the gateway to all this tragedy is the essential distortion of reality—one of the key signs of addictive disorder. This is why Cooper called cybersex the "crack cocaine" of sex addiction.[1]

People in all walks of life are experiencing problems with cybersex:

- the honor-roll college student whose cybersex activities caused him to flunk out of school and end up suicidal
- the attorney who became fascinated by images of young girls and struck up a relationship with an FBI agent posing as a thirteen-year-old girl as part of a sting operation
- the retiree who spent every morning downloading pornography and every afternoon e-trading, eventually draining all his retirement funds
- the single mother who felt so proud that she was able to work extra hours to support her family, not realizing that her eleven-year-old daughter spent almost twenty hours a week looking at adult pornography on the Net
- the wife of a successful physician who started innocently flirting with her husband's friends via e-mail and ended up having affairs with the majority of them

The list grows every day. And what these addicts have in common are distorted perceptions of reality and sufferance of severe consequences. The points that follow profile what happens to these people.

Compulsive Cybersex Involves Rapid Escalation of Amount and Variety of Sex

Problems for cybersex addicts often develop rapidly. Many of these addicts quickly find themselves doing the unthinkable. For example, a minister who was a trusted servant of his congregation turned on the very people he served and embezzled money from them to support his cybersex habit. It happened so quickly. It started off with just a membership to one or two clubs and escalated from there. The minister went from being a highly esteemed community leader to becoming someone he never imagined possible.

Escalation of Cybersex Use Becomes Obsessional with New Behaviors Becoming Quickly Fixated

Cybersex addicts can quickly become focused on new types of behavior in a very short amount of time—what has taken other sex addicts decades to develop before the advent of the Internet. For example, through the Internet, addicts can rapidly check out different chat rooms and discover new sexual practices that were never a part of their sexual repertoire. They may begin to explore and become fixated on specific topics such as women urinating, black heavy-breasted women, men over sixty, or hairless young men. Addicts become obsessed and can't stop thinking about cybersex. They begin to seek others who share their same interests through chat rooms and news groups.

Cybersex Addiction Involves Significant Relational Regression

With endless hours on the Net, little time exists for friends or family. Spare time becomes Internet time. Addicts regress developmentally as they become progressively more isolated. They lose intimacy as opposed to gaining it. Ironically, they begin to feel closer to people on the Net than people in their real lives. An example of this is a woman sitting in her home office transfixed on the computer screen while her kids are fighting outside and the house is in chaos. She's oblivious to

all that is going on with her family and home. She is so absorbed in the Internet that she has lost touch with reality. She
begins to neglect her family and experiences relational regres-
sion.

Compulsive Cybersex Accelerates Already Addictive Behavior

If sex addiction is already present, introducing cybersex is like
throwing gasoline on the flame. Sex addicts consistently report that their cyberactivities just facilitated what they were
already into. For example, if someone has a problem with
compulsive sex, the Net expands his or her ability to carry
that out. Cybersex creates a danger of relapse for those in recovery from sex addiction. The Internet allows addicts an opportunity to break down previous boundaries. For example,
they can view prostitutes online instead of soliciting prostitutes in person.

Compulsive Cybersex Can Result in Offline Sex Addiction

Some addicts start with cybersex and then escalate to other
behaviors. Cybersex becomes a catalyst to compulsive sex.
Addicts can easily find themselves aroused while using the
Internet and eventually seek real-life prostitutes both online
and offline.

The Computer and Internet Become Sexualized

The keyboard, specific Web sites, and even the sound of the
modem become eroticized. This becomes a problem for those
who must use a computer in their lives. For example, one man
became aroused just viewing the Yahoo Web site, knowing all

the sexually explicit Web sites it could access for him. Anything can become a turn-on, even images and sounds that would not typically be considered arousing. Even the sound of someone typing on a computer keyboard could be considered arousing to some.

The Internet is a great boon to humankind. It also has been a potent antidote to restrictive, antisexual attitudes in our culture, which themselves create obsession in people. It has created a new freedom to explore human sexuality as opposed to relying on negative sexual attitudes and myths. The problem is that some people start down a path they would never have pursued were it not for the freedom of the Internet. And some people create their own nightmares. In order to understand how that downfall develops for all sex addicts (not just cybersex addicts), we need to explore how people are aroused.

THE AROUSAL TEMPLATE

Arousal occurs in the brain. The brain is a constellation of circuits that conducts electricity through a maze of chemical interactions based on connectors called neurons. Scientists and physicians refer to neurochemical "cascades" that are virtual rivers of energy. Another name for them is neuropathways. There are three basic neuropathways in sex. The most primitive one, and the one that evolved first, causes us to be sexually aroused by others. After all, to be attracted to others is a survival function because it adds to the gene pool. However, as we evolved, it became more functional to pair up to protect offspring. Two more neuropathways then emerged. First, there evolved a neurochemistry to romance that involves great arousal, intensity, and obsession. It actually creates a period of "insanity" in which dopamine levels go up and serotonin levels decline. And second, an attachment neuropathway emerged allowing us to bond with one another. Some of the most powerful neurochemicals in the brain are generated by this bonding process. At times, all three of these neuropathways work together and at other times they conflict. But as sex researcher Helen Fisher observes, most cultures find it most functional to be involved with one person at a time.[2]

Neuropathways mobilize powerful chemicals that exist in the brain. Early sex researchers noted the overlap between the sexual neuropathways and the neuropathways of addiction. The famous Johns Hopkins University researcher John Money hypothesized in the early 1980s that the sexual neuropathways could be the "prototype" of all addictions. Access to the neuropathways comes through what Money termed a "lovemap" that every one of us carries inside. Between the ages of five and eight, most of us already have formed this map about what is sexually arousing to us. It serves as a template with which we decide whether a specific situation is arousing—and then we act on that template.[3]

Problems occur when that template or map becomes distorted. Minimal distortion occurs when a family will not talk about sex or casts a negative judgment about anything sexual. Early sexual experiences, especially if they involve shame or fear, can also distort beliefs about sex. Physical and sexual abuse can have a profound effect on what Money termed a "vandalization" of a person's lovemap. The tragic result can be that the person may become aroused in ways that are self-destructive or not functional. Here are some examples:

- A girl reads the sexually explicit magazines in her father's pornography collection and becomes convinced that that is how to get a man's attention. As an adult, she acts like a woman in those magazines to attract the attention of the opposite sex.

- A boy learns about sex looking at women wearing lingerie in department store catalogs. He becomes fixated on lingerie and discovers lingerie Web sites. He also becomes sexually involved with a woman who works for a lingerie company. He is arrested for breaking into people's homes and taking lingerie.

- A girl's mother is married four times. One of the girl's stepfathers molests her and her siblings. She approaches her mother about this. Her mother does nothing. At age fifteen she is involved with a "swinging club" of parents. At that same age she is allowed to have boys stay overnight. As she grows older and gets married, she has affairs and discloses this to her husband. He acts as if it does not matter to him, just like her mom acted toward her.

- A boy has surgery on his testicle. His mother is a nurse and tends to his wounds. On the Internet he discovers sites that feature old women and young boys together. He becomes fixated with "elder erotica."

- A mother pulls her son's pants down in front of her friends to show them his genitals, at which they all laugh and joke. As an adult, he ends up exhibiting himself and being humiliated.

- As punishment, a young girl had to take off her clothes in order to be beaten in front of her siblings. As an adult, she could only achieve an orgasm if a man was hurting her.

Notice in these examples that some of the situations were intentional abuse, some were inadvertent, and some were accidental. But all these incidents became incorporated into what was arousing for these children as adults. These experiences were integrated into the arousal template. When sex becomes addictive, it's often because this template, as well as the total belief system of the addict, is distorted.

Often there is a story or scenario embedded in the template that becomes replicated. But many things can be part of that arousal, including

- feelings that have become eroticized in some way. For example, anger that is acted out in a sexual way can become eroticized rage.
- locations such as hotel rooms, shopping centers, beaches, parks, certain parts of town, or specific cities or countries.
- objects such as automobiles, computer keyboards, sex toys, school uniforms, lingerie, or shoes.
- processes such as smoking, urination, violence, or degradation.
- body types or body parts including muscles, wrinkles, stretch marks, and fat.
- partner characteristics such as age, marital status, or personality types or traits (vulnerable, unreachable, hurtful, or unavailable).
- ethnic groups such as Asian women, African American men, or Hispanic gay men.
- courtship stages where elements of courtship become obsessive, such as when attraction turns into voyeurism and dysfunctional courtship beliefs such as "all women tease" or "men only want sex."

Successful recovery usually involves addicts and coaddicts understanding clearly how their arousal templates function. Usually this means understanding overarching stories or fantasies, making sense of how their lovemaps became "vandalized," and being able to discern healthy from unhealthy arousal.

Cybersex has the potential for further template distortion. People have parts of their sexual history in which things are unresolved, that is, "unfinished" parts about which they remain curious or interested. As they grow older, people do not have as much access to ways of exploring unresolved parts of their sexuality. The Net, however, opens the possibilities of exploring with little or no risk. And so people do, and encounter material that accesses those unresolved parts of themselves. This process can become very compelling. Cybersex addicts will talk of intrusive "burned-in" images that keep coming up in their consciousness. They become consumed with these images in much the same way abuse victims cannot stop thinking about when they were hurt. The images seem to be "burned-in" and difficult to filter. This is usually because that image somehow accessed the person in a profound way. Usually it is about the arousal template and something unresolved.

Computers and the Internet can easily accelerate the process. For example, marketing loops on pornography sites are designed to bombard the viewer with many images within a few seconds of entering a site. The intent is to appeal to something specific within that person. Pop-up screens and hyperlinks automatically link one pornographic site to the next. If these sites manage to hit a vulnerable area or stimulate something unknown, arousal templates become altered. Many recovering persons report how they found something on the Net that they never even knew about and how it quickly became obsessional. And consider the impact of instant messaging; romance junkies can "court" four or five people simultaneously without each being aware of the others. The stimulation can be more information than neuropathways were designed to handle. Once you understand that, cybersex as the "crack cocaine" of sex addiction makes sense.

Cybersex becomes the great accelerator of the addictive process. But it is not alone. Another key component of the addict's system is the larger network of family and loved ones who are part of the addictive cycle. Their behavior, too, emerges in patterns that interact and cycle. The family's participation in the addict's world is the focus of the next chapter.

CHAPTER 4

The Family and the Addict's World

□   □   □

> James Cermak's attorney, Fred Bruno, argued that sentencing
> Cermak for each sex offense would be like sentencing an alco-
> holic for each drink he takes.
>
> —*Minneapolis Tribune*, January 20, 1982

News of the Cermak brothers grabbed the public's attention
for almost a year. Few tales were as grim as the unfolding
story of their sexual abuse of a large number of children from
their rural Minnesota town. The children included all of their
own children plus others from the community. Most were ele-
mentary- or junior-high-age youngsters, the youngest being
the three-year-old son of James Cermak. Both brothers, James
and John, were sentenced to forty years in prison, neither
being eligible for parole for at least twenty-six years.

Central to the Cermaks' activities was playing something
they called "the game." Done in their homes or hotel rooms,
"the game" started with the children sitting on a bed in a circle
with no clothes on. They were then asked to perform sexual
acts with one another. The game concluded with the Cermaks
being sexual with the children, including oral intercourse.
Children were told they were "naughty" if they did not play
and were threatened with physical violence if they resisted.

The number of children involved, the sexual violation and

the emotional vulnerability of the children, and the cruelty of the Cermak brothers generated public outrage. The brothers' parents, Stanley and Alice, protested that the children had been "programmed" by the prosecuting attorney and denied the allegations. Yet more than 130 pieces of evidence were introduced, including about 70 instant photographs of the children in obscene poses or performing sexual acts. Even the Cermak brothers acknowledged the depth of the tragedy. John Cermak was so remorseful that suicidal feelings were a problem. James Cermak told the judge, "I'm sorry for the things I have done and I'm only twenty-six years old and I definitely need help."[1]

Hardly had public outrage started to subside when shocking new revelations appeared in the media. Beverly and Jillayne Cermak, the wives of James and John, were also being charged with child rape. They had both played "the game." Beverly was accused of having sex with seven children and forcing them to perform sex acts with other children over a two-and-a-half-year period. Jillayne was charged with eighteen counts of sexual abuse of children, nine of which were counts of first-degree criminal sexual conduct. Both Jillayne and Beverly were accused of aiding and abetting their husbands.

The Cermak story is classic if extreme: the denial of the grandparents in their efforts to protect the family secrets, the seemingly unending series of disclosures that gave testimony to how sexual obsession prevailed in the lifestyle of the family, the profound feelings of remorse, regret, and helplessness of the offenders, the loyalty of children who did not wish to testify against their parents, spouses who collaborated, and a public who chose to see the tragic series of events as isolated, bizarre, and unique.

Sexual compulsiveness, like all addictions, rests in a complex web of family relationships. The Cermaks are unique only in the degree to which their addiction escalated and the amount of publicity they got. Among the Cermak tragedies is the fact that each of the children involved has a high potential for participating in an addictive relationship as an adult. This chapter and the following are designed to show how the sexual addiction is a family illness and to trace how the abuse of children makes them vulnerable to addictive relationships. Most important will be to show the relationship of the family to the world of the addict as described in chapters 1, 2, and 3.

THE ROLE OF THE FAMILY

Sexual addiction, as a family illness, parallels almost every other emotional and addictive disorder. For the past twenty years professionals in many disciplines have been documenting the family as a "system"—regulated by rules and roles, understanding and misunderstanding. The family system has the capacity to sustain unity, establish the distance between family members, allow individual uniqueness, and produce organized effort. The family, above all, has a range of options available to maintain balance. Being balanced for family members makes them feel normal. Not always, but sometimes, this means keeping things the same even if they are painful.

Suicide, schizophrenia, alcoholism, runaways—all are part of the family epic. For example, in alcoholism, treatment of the spouse alone has been shown to promote recovery in the alcoholic. Now, throughout the ranks of specialists in addiction, treating the entire family is regarded as critical. It is recognized that the more that family members are involved, the higher the recovery rate. Moreover, spouses, parents, and children, by virtue of their participation in the family insanity, have a right to recovery for themselves.

Whatever the disorder, family members are often unaware

of their own pain. They very clearly do not understand their
contribution to the family drama. A sign of the family members' delusion is their deep-seated conviction that they had
little to do with it. If only that other person

- would stop drinking
- could control eating
- could keep his or her feet on the ground
- had not run away
- were not always depressed
- would get off the computer
- were not so obsessed with sex
- could manage life better
- would stop spending money
- were more responsible
- could keep a job
- would grow up and stop acting like a child

Then there would be no problems.

A more severe delusion is when the family does not even
acknowledge that there is a problem. Therein may be the ultimate tragedy of the Cermak grandparents, who protested that
the children were programmed by the prosecuting attorney.
By maintaining the public image of the family, the family
member can hold the pain at bay until the consequences come
crashing in. The ultimate revelation in the Cermak case came
when the public learned that James and John Cermak, the accused, had been victimized by their father. Both grandparents
were also accused of being sexual with their grandchildren.
Family denial appears to be accelerated in the sexual addiction because of the shame and moral connotations of sexual
behavior. In that sense, sexual addiction as a family dysfunction is different from other family illnesses. Yet the task
remains for each member of the family to search out his or her

individual part in the family predicament. All first efforts in understanding one's part in the family begin with the family in which one was raised. Part of acknowledging true powerlessness for both the addict and the concerned persons starts with the recognition that the roots of the addiction may, in fact, span generations.

Many of the stories throughout this book indicate the transmission of sexual addiction from one generation to the next. The question to answer now is how this transfer occurs.

There are four factors in a child's development that ultimately become part of the sexual addiction:

1. self-image—how children perceive themselves
2. relationships—how children perceive their relationships with others
3. needs—how children perceive their own needs
4. sexuality—how children perceive their own sexual feelings and needs

These perceptions ultimately become "core beliefs" central to the addictive system. They are conclusions that can govern choices and behaviors during the child's adult life. In this chapter, we will focus on how the process of developing core beliefs unfolds for the addict. In the next chapter, the evolving core beliefs of other family members will be examined.

Self-image and Relationships

Morris was an exhibitionist. He had initially started to expose himself as a teenager, but exposure remained only as an off-and-on problem until his early forties. Until then, he was involved in nudist clubs, in a few affairs, and with numerous prostitutes. The crisis for the family occurred when Morris started to expose himself to a neighbor woman next door.

Then he started to expose to passersby. The experience was extremely horrifying for the family, who had to suffer neighborhood outrage, police harassment, and the sale, at a loss, of their home of ten years. The more his wife, Linda, would try to control his behavior, the worse it became. With both involved in therapy and a Twelve Step group for sexual compulsiveness, and with their move providing a fresh start, Morris was able to redirect his life.

As a child, Morris was raised by his alcoholic father. His mother left them when he was six. While his father traveled, Morris was left at a boardinghouse run by two spinster sisters. He was the only child in the house, the rest of the residents being older men. The two sisters found numerous occasions to punish him with severe brutality. Punishment meant taking his clothes off and beating him, especially around the genital area. After these sessions the old men would comfort the boy by masturbating him to sleep.

The two sisters set up traps for Morris to guarantee "punishment" sessions. For example, knowing that the Saturday matineé ended at 3:00, they would tell the boy to return no later than 2:30. Obviously Morris would not be able to pass up the end of his movie and would arrive a half hour late. The punishment was, therefore, rationalized. The father would not believe the boy's stories, so Morris lived under these conditions from the age of six until he was ten and his father remarried. A significant part of Morris's therapy was to return to the small Illinois town in which these events took place and grieve over a lost childhood.

The story of Morris illustrates common antecedents to addiction. First, there is alcoholism in the family. Second, physical and emotional abuse accompany sexual abuse. Third, sexual experience is both humiliating and comforting. And fourth, the reality of the child is denied when the child's accounts of abuse are not taken seriously. All of these are potent contributors to the addiction, as we shall see.

By far the most important factor, however, is a sense of having been abandoned. From a child's point of view, "you can abuse me, humiliate me, exploit me, and even not believe me, but by far the worst is if you don't even want me." Fear of abandonment is a constant theme in all addictions, including alcoholism. Within the sexual addiction, it is especially powerful.

Abandonment has a thousand forms. Some forms are explicit, such as Morris's mother leaving him at age six and his dad traveling. In some cases certain events are interpreted as abandonment. Corky, for example, was a twenty-year-old exhibitionist who was also chemically dependent. His mother died when Corky was thirteen. He started exposing himself almost immediately, the first arrest happening only a few months after her death. An important part of his therapy came when he was able to connect his exhibitionism to how alone he felt when his mother died.

Even the threat of abandonment can be potent. Researchers H. Eist and A. Mandel describe how, within families where incest has occurred, "tremendous parental threats of abandonment were a most frequent technique employed by the parents to control or immobilize their children."[2] In writing about sexual compulsiveness, Julia Sherman has termed this phenomenon the "Coatlicue Complex," after the Aztec mother of the gods who symbolized "the power of life and death that each mother holds over her infant."[3] The sexual addiction receives its power from a fundamental concern for survival.

The first core belief of the addict is "I am basically a bad, unworthy person." Abandonment means being unwanted. The child can only conclude that being unwanted means being unworthy and bad.

A good example was Art, a twenty-seven-year-old chemically dependent man whose sexual addiction included multiple relationships, exhibitionism, voyeurism, obscene calls,
and eventually rape. When he was four years old, his mother
left and his alcoholic father remarried. His father was a sexual
addict and so were several uncles. Art writes in his autobiography about living with his stepmother:

> My brother and I were pretty regular brats and we took
> a lot of sadistic and humiliating treatment from our
> mother. One of her favorite punishments was tying us
> to chairs. Sometimes she'd make us wear diapers. We
> were old enough to be extremely mortified by it. She
> made my brother play outside like that once.
>
> Another fun thing my mother did to me was to dress
> me up like a girl. She put makeup on me and curlers in
> my hair and thought what a cute girl I would have made.
>
> Obviously, with three boys she must have wanted a
> girl, but what a crummy thing to do. I went along with
> it but I felt really embarrassed.
>
> I have a lot of hatred for women and a lot of it is
> from my mother. A lot of resentment came out—just
> that she wasn't my real mother. I guess I have some
> anger at my real mother for abandoning me even
> though I understand she tried to get custody.
>
> After she ran out of ways to punish us we had to sit
> and think of our own punishments. I spent a lot of time
> thinking of different ways to be punished. This is where
> I got a lot of my guilt and shame and when I learned to
> be self-punishing.

Note again the themes of abuse, punishment, and humiliation, as well as abandonment. The more prevalent these elements are, the more compelling the addiction.

A second core belief comes from the first core belief about the child being a bad person. Because of personal unworthiness, the child believes, "No one would love me as I am." Relationships with others become more tenuous the deeper this belief is. Children grow up believing that no one will accept them unconditionally. People will not be there; they cannot be trusted or depended on. If they do want a relationship, it is because they want something—not because they care. There will always be a price to pay. Minimally, there will be something that must be overlooked, ignored, or denied. To be close will mean to lose reality or integrity somehow. So intimacy is avoided. As the child grows up, a personal front or public image designed to look good shields the emerging adult from the searching gaze of others, which would lead to rejection.

Needs and Sexuality

Addicts report that as children they felt desperately lonely, lost, and unprotected. Not only was there a lack of nurturing, but also there was no one to show them how to take care of themselves or keep them from harm. Not being able to count on, depend upon, the adults in one's life to meet needs is a key element in addiction. As the child matures, there begins a search for that which is dependable—something that you can trust to make you feel better. Trust and dependency are the issues that determine personal strength and confidence or vulnerability to enslaving addiction. For in the lonely search for something or someone to depend on—which has already excluded parents—a child can start to find those things which always comfort, which always feel good, which always are there, and which always do what they promise. For some, alcohol and drugs are the answer. For others it is food. And there is always sex, which usually costs nothing and nobody else can regulate.

This choice stems from the addict's third core belief that is about needs: "My needs are never going to be met if I have to depend upon others." In healthy families, children have a deep sense that their parents care for them as opposed to abandoning them.

Healthy parenting includes touching, loving, affirming, and guiding. The child feels cared for even when struggling with rules and limits. Trust in one's self, as well as trust of others, emerges in that relationship.

When a child's exploration of sexuality goes beyond discovery to routine self-comforting because of the lack of human care, there is potential for addiction. Sex becomes confused with comforting and nurturing. Moreover, the assumption is made that everyone else feels and acts the same. Therefore, to feel secure means to be sexual.

Consequently, the child's relationships with people have the potential for being replaced with an addictive relationship with sexuality. Addiction is a relationship—a pathological relationship in which sexual obsession replaces people. And it can start very early. The final core belief of the addict emerges clearly: "Sex is my most important need."

The kinds of childhood situations described here are further complicated when the children are surrounded by negative rules, messages, and judgments about sex. When addicts and their spouses study their families of origin, they are flooded with memories of events where they were told that being sexual was bad or, worse, that they were bad for being sexual.

When children's primary source of comfort is sex and yet they are told by those whose judgments count the most that to be sexual is perverse, the conclusions they make about themselves are clear. They are unlikable. They need to hide that central part of themselves, which others will despise. Rather than repressing the sexual behaviors, they hide them or keep them secret. Needing to keep that central part of themselves secret adds to the pain and loneliness—which, in turn, creates a need for comfort, making the sexual fix that much more necessary. The fusion between sex and nurturing is cemented if the children are victims of sexual abuse. Level Two and Level Three addicts are almost always sexually abused as children. Parents, clergy, older siblings, relatives, physicians, friends, teachers, baby-sitters—a wide range of people have the potential of exploiting a child. Children learn from the important adults in their lives how to have a significant human relationship. Once a person has learned how to have a relationship with other people, then the sexual component can be added as an expression of a special relationship. If the parents or significant adults are sexual with the child, the young person will always have difficulty sorting out sexuality and relationship.

The Abuse Checklist, following on pages 104 and 105, is intended as a guide to help addicts identify sexual, physical, and emotional abuse that occurred in their childhoods.

A sexual addict exploring his early years can pick out the most blatant examples of victimization. There are, however, a number of factors that can obscure the victimization. For example, professionals such as clergy, physicians, teachers, and therapists who are sexual within the context of their profession are hard to detect if their intentions are not explicit. Thus, a child who feels "funny" about the physical exam he received decides that it was imagination. The feeling or intuition, however, may have been very accurate.

Sexual compulsivity also obscures victimization. Addicts consider any sexual contact as a victory. Addicts commonly discover, as they share their sexual history with other addicts,

The following checklist and worksheet will help you assess the extent to which you were abused in your own childhood experience. Read over each of the three categories of abuse (sexual, physical, emotional). Fill in the information in the spaces next to the items that apply to you.

FORM OF ABUSE	AGE
A. Sexual Abuse	
Suggestive flirtatiousness	_____
Propositioning	_____
Inappropriate holding, kissing	_____
Fondling of sexual parts	_____
Masturbation	_____
Oral sex	_____
Forceful sexual activity	_____
Other	_____
B. Physical Abuse	
Shoving	_____
Slapping, hitting	_____
Scratches, bruises	_____
Burns	_____
Cuts, wounds	_____
Broken bones, fractures	_____
Damage to organs	_____
Permanent injury	_____
Other	_____
C. Emotional Abuse	
Neglect	_____
Harassment, malicious tricks	_____
Blackmail	_____
Unfair punishments	_____
Cruel or degrading tasks	_____
Cruel confinement	_____
Abandonment	_____
Other	_____

Figure 4.1

CHECKLIST

For each type of abuse, record the information to the best of your memory:

Age: How old were you when it started?

Abusing Persons: Who abused you? Father, stepfather, mother, stepmother, adult relative, adult friend, adult neighbor, professional person, brother or sister, or stranger?

Frequency: How often did it happen? Daily, two to three times a week, weekly, monthly, or occasionally?

ABUSING PERSON   **FREQUENCY**

that many of their early sexual experiences were exploitive. They learn, for example, that for a fourteen-year-old boy to be sexual with a woman in her thirties is for him to be abused. Yet the boy doesn't identify this as abuse. When it feels good, it is hard to notice. From the addict's point of view as an adolescent, it was a "score."

One of the hardest barriers to overcome for addicts in understanding their own victimization is family loyalty. Children are incredibly loyal, even under the worst conditions. Not only parents, uncles, and cousins, but also even stepparents and family friends are not to be betrayed. These family bonds are reinforced by a rule that says, "The family takes care of its own problems." Like all victims, addicts have difficulty in breaking the family "secret" to others.

For those addicts who have experienced family sexual abuse, breaking the secret is the most explicit way to trace the transmission of the sexual addiction from one generation to the next.

One addict who, in addition to compulsive use of prostitutes and extramarital affairs, had been incestuous with two of his three sons, made a major breakthrough in recalling his own childhood. His father told him when he was a child that the doctor had asked that he manipulate his son's foreskin in order to ensure its flexibility when he became an adult. This manipulation led to frequent sexual contact between father and son. When the father's father (grandfather of the sons) was brought into therapy, he admitted that in fact he had not talked to the doctor, but had learned it from *his* father. How did the great-grandfather know? From his father. The special irony in all of this was that the addict had been circumcised.

Children do not have to be victimized in order to be affected by the victimization. A son who lives in the house in which his sisters are victimized is clearly at risk. Similarly, being in the presence of sexual compulsivity of any form has its impact and creates vulnerability to addiction. Addicts frequently discover that their behavior parallels that of their parents or relatives. The addict—as well as his spouse— absolutely needs to know if there were affairs or prostitutes or compulsive acting out in the preceding generations.

Sexual compulsivity in previous generations is usually a well-guarded secret. The addicts believe they are the only ones who are sexually compulsive, which increases their shame. What they do not know is that the judgment and neg- ative rules around sex originate in the obsession of the parent, who fears that the compulsivity he or she has experienced might happen to the child. Unwittingly, the parents' efforts to contain sexual activity add a key negative catalyst to the ad- diction, as the previous generation did.

The cosmic observer would have an epic spectacle of gener- ations of sexual addicts all lost in their own loneliness and com- pulsivity. Lonely as children, they are lonely as parents. Unable to admit they need help to make things different, they create the very same empty environment for their own children.

THE CORE BELIEFS OF THE ADDICT'S WORLD

All addicts can find elements of their sexual compulsiveness in their early years. Even if no overt experiences of abuse exist, the fundamental self-doubt and distrust of others lie waiting as potential factors in addiction. Examples of all four core beliefs can be identified in the addict's childhood. However, when the addiction takes over, an addict's life varies according to individual life experience. For some, the compulsiveness starts early, such as in the case of the young exhibitionist who started exposing himself right after his mother's death. For others, compulsiveness emerges full force in adult years, usually in response to stress and anxiety. For every addict the common denominator is the addictive system described in chapter 1. The addict's belief system lays the foundation for impaired thinking that supports the addictive cycle (preoccupation, ritualization, compulsive pattern of sex and behavior, depression). The resulting unmanageability and powerlessness confirm and deepen the core beliefs. At that point, when the belief system, including the core beliefs, is intensified, the addictive system becomes fully engaged.

The core beliefs that were part and parcel of the addict's growing up become central to the addict's world as an adult. Each core belief contributes to the disconnection between the interior world the addict experiences, with its pain and shame, and the exterior image the addict projects to keep the secret world safe. The addict lives in constant personal "jeopardy," dreading the moment when the secret world will be unmasked. The addict becomes more isolated as the secret life grows. Family and friends become more peripheral. Loved ones struggle with the increasing alienation, as well as a mounting number of discrepancies between what the addict says and does. They cannot penetrate into the addict's secret world. Each core belief adds to the barriers protecting the internal world.

The belief "I am basically a bad, unworthy person" structures the emotional foundations of the addict's world. Addicts conclude from their family experiences that they are not worthwhile persons. Feelings of inadequacy and failure predominate. Addicts even see humiliation and degradation as justified or deserved. The desperate struggle around sexual compulsivity absolutely confirms this belief and enhances feelings of low self-worth. Addicts are committed to hiding the secret reality of their addiction at all costs because of their unworthiness. Yet the addiction guides almost all behavior and decisions.

Addicts create a front of "normalcy" to hide their sense of inadequacy. They may even appear grandiose and full of exaggerated self-importance. The front contrasts with actions that appear degrading or self-defeating or both. Others see decisions or behaviors as irrational, unfathomable, or even self-destructive, but not "normal."

Close friends and family members become angry and frustrated with the addict's egocentric quality, especially when there is insensitivity to others. They are troubled at what looks like destructive or curious behavior that does not fit the image the addict projects.

The belief "No one would love me as I am" also sustains the secret world. Addicts continue to believe that everyone would abandon them if the truth were known. Consequently, they have a constant fear of being vulnerable or dependent on others. Addicts perceive their behavior as so bad that everything that goes wrong becomes their fault. Addicts assume responsibility for all the pain in loved ones. Honest guilt and remorse cannot be expressed because that would require honesty about behavior. Addicts progressively become more isolated from normal contact with family and friends.

Yet addicts create the image of being in charge of life and in no need of help. They appear unaffected by any problems, but will often do extreme or indulgent things as if making up for something. No explanation is offered, however. Some addicts may continue to be charming and sociable, but all addicts become "unreachable" personally as they close off all avenues of vulnerability.

Significant persons in the addict's life start to feel cut out, pushed away, useless, neglected, and unnecessary. They become confused: the addict makes seemingly generous gestures, but lacks any personal warmth or presence. The family and friends feel angry, hurt, and rejected in response to the addict's contradictory behavior.

"My needs are never going to be met if I have to depend upon others" is the belief that provides the addiction with its driving power. The survival needs of the child are transformed into the desperation of the addict's interior world. Basically, addicts feel unloved and unlovable, which means their needs will be unmet. The resulting rage becomes internalized as depression, resentment, self-pity, and even suicidal feelings. Because they have no confidence that others will love them, addicts become calculating, strategizing, manipulative, and ruthless. Rules and laws are designed for people who are lovable. Those who are unlovable have to survive in other ways.

The addict's rage about unmet needs in the past prevents the possibility of expressing needs now, because addicts anticipate that they will be rejected. Consequently, addicts appear not to want or need anything at a human level. They are purposely unclear about their intentions in relationships, which makes for a kind of seductive behavior; that is, they try to be affirmed or cared for without expressing that they need it so they will not be rejected. Addicts make extensive efforts to show how respectable and law-abiding they are.

As consequences to the addiction begin to emerge, those who are close start to see the double life, the Jekyll and Hyde, in the addict's world. The addict's ups and downs remain difficult to understand. Worse, family and friends begin to distrust and disbelieve the addict. Things appear to be so smooth, yet the intuition is that they are not. Inconsistencies between the addict's public and private lives confirm these intuitions.

The belief that makes sexual obsession the focus of the addiction is "Sex is my most important need." The addict continues to confuse nurturing and sex. Support, care, affirmation, and love are all sexualized. Absolute terror of life without sex combines with feelings of unworthiness for having such intense sexual desires. Sexual activity never meets the need for love and care, but it continues to be seen as the only avenue. The addict has a high need to control all situations in an effort to guarantee sex. Yet there is a secret fear of being sexually out of control. Addicts promise themselves to stop or limit sexual behavior because of this fear.

Sexual obsession pervades the addict's lifestyle and behavior. The addict makes the maximum effort to ensure all possible sexual opportunities. All levels of addictive behavior directly reflect the need to control sexual access. In other words, multiple affairs, prostitution, exhibitionism, voyeurism, incest, rape, and so on, have in common the goal of protecting "the source of supply." Seeking degrading or humiliating sexual experiences simply extends internal feelings of unworthiness. However, addicts profess extreme sexual propriety, even to the extent of moral self-righteousness about sexual matters. Cover-ups, lies, and deceptions are made to conceal personal sexual behavior.

The addict's protestations of high sexual morality are like a smoke screen, obscuring the impact of sexual obsession. Friends and family tend to reject suspicions of sexual compulsivity because of the addict's "values." However, as evidence of powerless behavior and unmanageability mounts, these persons are confused because they do not know what to believe. In addition, they do not wish to intervene in something so personal. Finally, the distance and lack of personal connection take their toll. Since few feel close enough to say anything, they choose the other option, which is to withdraw.

The following chart, The World of the Sexual Addict, summarizes how the core beliefs learned in childhood continue to influence the interior and exterior portions of the addict's world, as well as the family members and friends of the addict.

The sexual addiction clearly has its roots in the family life of the addict. The role of the family does not end there, however. The family continues to play an integral part in the ad-

---

THE WORLD OF THE

CORE BELIEF 1
SELF-IMAGE: I am basically a bad,
unworthy person.

Interior World

Addicts conclude from their family experiences that they are not worthwhile persons. Feelings of inadequacy and failure predominate. Addicts often see humiliation and degradation as justified or deserved. The desperate struggle around sexual compulsivity absolutely confirms this belief and enhances feelings of low self-worth. Addicts are committed to hiding the secret reality of their addiction at all costs because of their unworthiness. Yet the addiction guides almost all behavior and decisions.

Exterior World

Addicts create a front of "normalcy" to hide their sense of inadequacy. They may even appear grandiose and full of exaggerated self-importance. As consequences to behaviors emerge, the front contrasts with actions that seem to be degrading or self-defeating or both. Others see decisions or behaviors as irrational, incomprehensible, or even self-destructive, but not "normal."

Family and Friends

Close friends and family members become angry and frustrated with the addicts' egocentricity, especially when there is insensitivity to others. Not knowing the interior world of an addict, they are troubled by what looks like destructive or curious behavior that does not fit the image the addicts project.

Figure 4.2

dictive system. This part is called coaddiction. When family members become so involved in one addiction that they participate in the illness, they are called coaddicts. They are the focus of the next chapter.

SEXUAL ADDICT

CORE BELIEF 2
RELATIONSHIPS: No one would love me
as I am.

Interior World	Addicts believe that everyone would abandon them if the truth were known. They have a constant fear of being dependent on others. Addicts perceive their sexual behavior as so bad that everything becomes their "fault." Addicts assume responsibility for all the pain in loved ones. Honest guilt and remorse cannot be expressed because that would require honesty about behavior. Addicts become progressively more isolated.
Exterior World	Addicts create the image of being in charge of life and in no need of help. They appear unaffected by any problem, but will often do extreme or indulgent things as if making up for something. No explanation is offered, however. Some addicts may continue to be charming and sociable, but all addicts become "unreachable" personally as they close off all avenues of vulnerability.
Family and Friends	Significant persons in the addicts' lives start to feel pushed away, useless, neglected, and unnecessary. They become confused at seemingly generous gestures, but in the absence of any personal warmth or presence. Anger and hurt accumulate with a sense of abandonment in reaction to the addicts' contradictory behavior.

CORE BELIEF 3
NEEDS: My needs are never going to be met
if I have to depend upon others.

Interior World

Addicts feel unloved and unlovable, which means other people cannot be depended on to love them, so their needs will not be met. The resulting rage becomes internalized as depression, resentment, self-pity, and even suicidal feelings. Because they have no confidence in others' love, addicts become calculating, strategizing, manipulative, and ruthless. Rules and laws are made for people who are lovable. Those who are unlovable survive in other ways.

Exterior World

Addicts' rage about unmet needs in the past prevents the possibility of expressing needs now because they anticipate being rejected. Addicts appear not to want or need anything. They are purposely unclear about their intentions in relationships and are thus seductive in behavior, i.e., they try to be affirmed or cared for without expressing that they need it so they will not risk rejection. Addicts make extensive efforts to show how respectable and law-abiding they are.

Family and Friends

Those who are close start to see the double life, the Jekyll and Hyde, in the addicts' worlds. The addicts' ups and downs remain difficult to understand. Worse, distrust and disbelief in the addicts begin. Things appear to be so smooth, yet the intuition is that they are not. Inconsistencies between the addicts' public and private lives confirm these intuitions.

Figure 4.2 *(Continued)*

CORE BELIEF 4
SEXUALITY: Sex is my most important need.

Interior World

Addicts confuse nurturing and sex. Support, care, affirmation, and love are all sexualized. Absolute terror of life without sex combines with feelings of unworthiness for such intense sexual desires. Sexual activity never meets the need for love and care, but continues to be seen as the only avenue to meeting those needs. Addicts have a high need to control all situations in an effort to guarantee sex. Yet there is a secret fear of being sexually out of control. Addicts promise themselves to stop or limit sexual behavior because of this fear.

Exterior World

Sexual obsession pervades lifestyle and behavior. Addicts make maximum effort to ensure all possible sexual opportunities. Addicts at all levels of addictive behavior feel the need to control sexual access; that is, addicts involved in prostitution, exhibitionism, voyeurism, incest, etc., have in common the goal of protecting the "source of supply." Seeking degrading or humiliating sexual experiences simply extends internal feelings of unworthiness. Addicts publicly profess extreme sexual propriety, however, even to the extent of moral self-righteousness about sexual matters. Cover-ups, lies, and deceptions are made to conceal personal sexual behavior.

Family and Friends

The addicts' protestations of high sexual morality obscure the impact of sexual obsession on friends and families. Close family and friends tend to reject suspicions of sexual compulsivity because of the addicts' "values." As evidence of powerlessness over behavior and unmanageability mounts, these persons become confused, not knowing what to believe. In addition, they do not wish to intervene in something so personal. Since they don't feel close enough to become involved, they choose the other option, which is to withdraw.

CHAPTER 5

Coaddiction

◘ ◘ ◘

> Ruth Coe, the mother of convicted rapist, Frederick Coe, was
> charged Friday with hiring a man she did not know was an
> undercover police officer to kill the prosecutor who tried her
> son and the judge who sentenced him to life in prison.
>
> —*Spokane Review*, November 21, 1981

The plight of Ruth Coe is a tragic example of the family illness
that affects those who care for the sexually compulsive. Her
son, Frederick Coe, was accused of being the "South Hill
rapist." Thirty-seven rapes were attributed to this rapist, who
employed a highly ritualized strategy of following women as
they left buses to walk to their homes. Coe was given life plus
seventy-five years on conviction for four of the rapes. During
the trial, Ruth Coe gained a certain notoriety for her testimony. She had elaborate alibis for her son, including a description of how she and her son had searched "together" for
the real South Hill rapist by following buses. The testimony
and her attempt at violent revenge create a profile of a woman
in profound pain about her son.

The tragedy of the Coe family was intensified by the fact
that Gordon Coe, the father, was the highly respected manag-
ing editor of the *Spokane Daily Chronicle*, one of the two metropolitan papers. Among the issues that emerged was whether

the press, particularly the rival *Spokane Review*, handled the case so sensationally that it prejudiced the trial of Fred Coe. Closely related was the issue of whether Ruth Coe was a victim of police entrapment. The heightened publicity obscured the very real pain and powerlessness of the Coe family.

Ruth Coe at the age of sixty-one was still active, aggressive, and attractive. She had distinguished herself in her college teaching as well as community activities. She clearly had violated her own value system in offering the undercover agent money. The psychologist who examined her reported her to be a woman in "deep grief." While Ruth Coe may or may not be a coaddict, grief and addiction have something in common: denial. One of the first reactions of a grieving person is the denial of the loss of the loved one. The loss of relationship because of addictive involvement generates all those basic human processes involved at separation: hope, denial, anger, despair, and loneliness. A grieving person resolves pain by acknowledging the loss and reconnecting with others. Losing a loved one to addiction, however, has the potential of keeping one stuck in the early stages of grief and never coming to resolution. The addict is still present in one's life even though the loss of the relationship is real.

Therein is the bind of the "coaddict," or the loved one or friend who becomes so involved in the life of the addict that he or she truly starts to participate in the same impaired mental processes of the addict. As "courtship goes awry" for the addict, the grief cycle for the loved one also becomes distorted. By definition, the addict replaces normal human relationships with sexual compulsiveness. Loved ones feel the loss, try to deny it, and become angry, feeling despair and sometimes hope. The coaddicts' efforts to restore the relationship are not only ineffective, they can intensify and deepen the addictive system for the addict. To compound the tragedy,

coaddicts will take actions which are self-destructive, degrading, or even profound violations of their own values. Family
members, as coaddicts, become part of the problem. Hence,
the prefix *co-*.

Ruth Coe maintained that her son was innocent. Publicly,
she was regarded as a mother who was attempting to protect
her son. Her attempt to hire someone to kill the judge and
prosecutor who sent her son to prison clarified for everyone
her lack of reality about her son's actions. Coaddicts will go to
extreme lengths to preserve the exterior world of the addict.
By their actions they enter the insanity of their own interior
coaddictive world.

The story of Beth illustrates well how the coaddict will distort reality in response to the addiction. Beth's parents were
alcoholic. As a child she did everything possible to look good
or be good. The violence and punishment were so great in her
family that she went to any extent to avoid conflict. Her extra
efforts at school, her extracurricular activities, and her jobs
served many purposes. She was away from home as much as
possible, she did not get into trouble, and she received attention for doing well. Although competent, Beth felt inadequate
most of the time. She believed she had to prove herself over
and over.

Men were a special problem. Beth was attractive but saw
herself as homely. She did not trust the advances of men.
Sexual experiences were disappointing since Beth always felt
exploited, until she met Gene. Beth saw Gene as the ideal man
for her. Besides being attractive, Gene also came from an alcoholic home. In fact, part of their initial attraction was that they
agreed they would never do what their parents had done.
Beth felt secure that, even though Gene drank, he had been
hurt as she was and would not become an alcoholic. Beth was
flattered by Gene's attention, given his previous involvement

with a number of different women. When he broke off an engagement with another woman, she truly felt chosen. In short, Beth saw him as the perfect male.

Beth's first question about Gene's faithfulness to her came about three months after their marriage. Gene had lost his wedding band. Since they were short on money, they did not replace it. Gene's story about the loss of the ring was plausible, yet she was bothered by it. Her secret fear was that she might not be sufficiently attractive, competent, and interesting to keep a man.

Two events accentuated that fear. About a year after they were married, Beth saw Gene in a park with another woman. Upon confronting Gene with having an affair, she separated from him for three months. Ultimately, Gene convinced her that it was a meaningless mistake and that they should start over again. The second event occurred shortly after the birth of their second child. Beth discovered another affair, about which she was intensely jealous. The combination of Gene's remorse and the burden of two little ones convinced Beth to make the best of it.

Gene was finally arrested for exhibitionism. He was not prosecuted, but it created quite a stir in the neighborhood. Beth was shocked and crushed, but this event was only the beginning. A neighbor friend who had heard about Gene came over. She asked if Beth had trouble getting baby-sitters. In fact, Beth had begun to wonder if their two children had become monsters, since all the regular sitters seemed to be "too busy." The neighbor suggested that she talk to the girls again and find out why they would not come. Beth coaxed the girls into admitting that Gene had, in fact, molested two of them on the way home. He had exposed himself to another while she was baby-sitting his children. Beth asked that they tell no one, that she would take care of it.

When confronted, Gene had a story for each instance, including the exposure; he said he went to the shower "not realizing the children and the sitter were around." She did not believe him but acted as if she did. Somehow she felt it was her fault for not meeting his sexual needs.

Beth became preoccupied with Gene's sexual obsessiveness. She only hired boy sitters. She would throw out his *Playboy* and *Penthouse* magazines. She watched him constantly to see if he was "rubbernecking" as attractive women went by. She became distant and cold. Her criticisms of Gene were harsh and judgmental. She often thought of leaving. She even thought of having affairs in retaliation.

In addition, Gene's drinking was becoming a problem. Beth found herself reacting to Gene in much the same way she had reacted to her parents. She became very active in the community, the children's schools, and her part-time job. She found living with Gene easier when it was "as if two ships were passing in the night." The drinking was bothersome, but Gene's sexual involvements were terrifying.

The last straw came one day when Beth called an old friend she had not seen in a long while. She became instantly aware that something was wrong. Asking her friend to be candid, Beth was not prepared for her story. Amid sobs and hesitations, her friend reminded her of a party to which the three of them had gone. Beth was dropped off. Gene drove the friend home. He walked her to her apartment and invited himself in. He made advances. When she resisted, he forcibly raped her. The friend explained that she did not think anyone would believe her. She had allowed him in and even thought she might have been responsible, since both of them had been drinking and flirting earlier at the party.

Beth was furious. Gene did not deny her friend's story. In fact, he told Beth that he felt really bad about the whole thing

and knew it was because of the drinking. The timing was incredible, since Gene's employer had just that day told Gene he
had to go in for a screening for alcoholism. Beth was dumb-
founded. She knew that Gene had a problem with drinking—
but the real problem was sex. Gene went to treatment partly
out of his shame about the revelation of Beth's friend. During
treatment, however, the program staff quickly helped Gene
and Beth to realize there were two addictions present. Beth
was obsessed with one and had been blind to the other.

Gene discovered in treatment that his sexual compulsivity
did not start with his marriage. Gene had brought to the marriage a complete fusion of sex and relationship. His obsessiveness went back to grade school, when he would sneak out
regularly at night, climb a tree, and watch a neighbor lady undress. He also had been sexually abused, starting at the age of
six by a baby-sitter. He even remembered a series of abusive
events in his parochial high school with friends, teachers, and
priests. One priest, in fact, regularly fondled Gene's genitals
during confession while explaining how masturbation was a
sin. He would say, "You know you are not supposed to use
this," as Gene would become aroused. That event pictured for
Gene what his youth was about—a double message about humiliation and excitement he never outgrew.

Like most addicts, Gene discovered that marriage did not
change his compulsiveness. Within three months of marrying
Beth he was involved with other women. He did love Beth,
and he did not even like the women with whom he was involved. The woman Beth saw in the park was someone Gene
really hated but would have sex with. With the separation,
Gene vowed never to be sexual again with anyone outside the
marriage. His promises to Beth had the ring of sincerity,
rooted in his commitment to change. Yet it was only a matter
of time before he was involved again. As repeated efforts to

stop failed and as his sexual behavior extended to exhibition-ism, Gene's profound discouragement about himself in-creased. The presence of children in his family simply added to the pain. Gene experienced what every addict who is also a parent experiences—to look at his children and wonder what they would think if they knew.

In treatment, Beth realized that her history with Gene re-vealed a consistent process in which she sacrificed her own identity—giving up a part of herself in order to stay in the re-lationship. This process included a range of strategies:

- disregarding her own intentions
- overlooking behavior that hurt her deeply
- covering up behavior that she despised
- appearing cheerful when she was hurting
- avoiding conflict to keep up appearances
- being disrespected repeatedly
- allowing her own standards to be compromised
- faulting herself for the family's problems
- believing she had no options

Everything Beth did was similar to what she had done to sur-vive as a child in an alcoholic family.

Beth's loss of self also paralleled the loss Gene suffered. Gene's life had been taken over by addiction. Beth, too, was caught in a process beyond her control—a process in which her reactions made the situation worse. Beth was truly a coaddict.

THE COADDICTIVE SYSTEM

The coaddictive system parallels the process of the addictive system. Coaddiction starts with fundamental or core beliefs about one's self, relationships, needs, and sexuality. These beliefs generate impaired thinking that distorts reality and fosters coaddictive behavior. This is behavior by which the coaddict attempts to change the addict, but which in reality contributes to the addiction. Coaddictive behavior adds to the unmanageability of the family members' lives. When the unmanageable consequences confirm the core beliefs, the co-addictive system grows and perpetuates itself. Each part of the system reinforces the others.

THE COADDICTIVE SYSTEM

Figure 5.1

The belief system again is key. Cultural and family messages affect what the child holds to be true. In many ways, the coaddict's core beliefs are the same as the addict's. Beth's belief about her basic undesirability limited her relationship possibilities. In order to survive and have her needs met, she felt she had to pretend that everything in the relationship was acceptable when it was not. The same sense of abandonment that addicts experience in their lives exists for coaddicts. A complete discussion of coaddicts' core beliefs appears later in this chapter. At this point the reader only needs to see the central role of the belief system. Since the belief system filters the reality of the coaddict, impaired thinking results.

First, there is *denial*. At its most subtle, denial is dismissing your own intuitions. At its most blatant, it is overlooking what is right in front of you. Both Ruth Coe and Beth had clear indicators that there was a serious problem but chose not to see it. One incestuous father used to have an elaborate ritual of making a special bed for his daughters late at night. He would get his daughters out of bed, take them to the extra bed, be sexual with them, and throw the sheets in the wash. During the eight years that this was a weekly occurrence, the mother never voiced any curiosity about where the extra sheets came from.

Denial is usually supported by extensive *rationalization*. Beth always had sound reasons to dismiss her feelings and reality. She even assured herself that if she and Gene were making love on a regular basis, things must be all right. Sometimes the family member's logic just does not make sense to outsiders. Ruth Coe faced that with the jury who convicted her son. He was accused of using colored transparencies to make his car license plates appear to be out-of-state plates. Her explanation was that he had used it to protect his personalized plates—which he no longer had. Moreover, she thought it was so fashionable she wanted him to do it for her car.

Grandiosity and *inadequacy* are flip sides of the same coin for the family members. Because they feel their own "failings" so deeply (inadequacy), they feel responsible for other people's actions (grandiosity). For example, "If only I had been more sexual, he would not have to do this." It is grandiose for the wife to assume responsibility for her husband's sexuality. She does so because she feels inadequate. It works the same way with all members of the family: "If only I had been a better child, parent, brother, or sister."

Perhaps the most damaging dynamics of the impaired thinking are *blame* and *judgment*. The coaddict judges the addict as the source of all the family's problems. Blaming the addict protects the coaddict from the vulnerability of telling the addict about personal hurts and fears. There is absolute safety in blame.

In healthy relationships, intimacy becomes possible when people accept the risk of rejection and reveal their internal struggles. Such self-disclosure between partners

- indicates trust
- affirms the other person
- takes responsibility for one's own actions and feelings
- shares common problems
- interrupts the addictive system

Blame, however, builds barriers instead of intimacy because it

- indicates distrust
- lowers self-worth
- builds defensiveness
- denies personal responsibility
- prevents efforts to work on common problems
- intensifies the addictive system

Blame, denial, secrecy, grandiosity, and rationalization together shield the coaddict's internal feelings of fear, hopelessness, and inadequacy. A person who is grieving the loss of the original relationship with the addict may refuse to accept reality, become angry and blaming, or even start to bargain with the addict. The coaddict wishes to stave off the pain that admitting the loss would bring. Similarly, the coaddict distorts reality in order to preserve the relationship. Even the most self-righteous blame preserves the coaddict's connection because by preoccupation with the addict's problems the coaddict can remain involved.

Preoccupation with the addict's sexual behavior bridges the gap between impaired thinking and coaddictive behavior. The coaddict's obsession with whether the addict is acting out or not obscures the coaddict's self-awareness. The desperate concentration pushes loneliness, pain, and vulnerability aside.

Preoccupation with the addict's problems leads to *controlling behavior* on the part of the spouse, parent, or significant other. When Beth threw out her husband's magazines, she was acting like the spouse of the alcoholic who pours booze down the drain. Neither one is effective in controlling addiction. Family members' efforts to control are rooted in the grandiose thinking that they can do something about shaping up the addict. Overt efforts to control include watching the addict, demanding accountability for all time spent, not trusting the addict to act responsibly, and even setting traps for the addict. These efforts are intensified by self-righteous criticism, blame, and judgment. The family tries to prove that the addict is the bad person and needs to change. The addict receives the message. (There is no other conclusion, given the addict's core beliefs.)

The coaddict uses the sexual relationship between them as one of the chief methods to control the addict. Controlling sex comes from the coaddict's preoccupation with the sexual behavior of the addict. Sexual manipulations include

- withdrawing sex as a punishment
- having sex as a reward
- threatening sex with others to create jealousy in the addict
- having sex with others to retaliate
- acting or dressing sexy to gain attention
- being sexual with the addict to prevent the addict from being sexual with others

In the short run, the coaddict can manipulate the sexual obsession of the addict. In the long run, the coaddict simply provides proof for the addict's belief that the most important need cannot be predictably met.

Enabling, in contrast to controlling, stems from denial and rationalization. Covering up for the addict, protecting him or her from consequences, and keeping silent about personal concerns are the behavioral ingredients of enabling. It involves a fundamental dishonesty that entails the insane denial of what one knows to be true. Beth often took the consequences for Gene. The paradox is that she could only do that by assuming she could change Gene.

Participation in secrecy clearly enables the addict's illness. When Beth asked the baby-sitters not to tell anyone, she, too, entered a double life. Beth was acting on two myths. The first was that all problems are to be solved within the family. The second was the conviction that she could control or stop the addiction. The efforts of the family members end up fueling or enabling the addiction, not stopping it. The veil of secrecy around the addictive behavior prevents outside feedback from restoring to the addict and family members a true grasp of reality. When Beth's neighbor confronted her, she was asking Beth to face up to a real problem, not bury it.

In fact, both the coaddictive behaviors, controlling and enabling, rest in the assumption that the coaddict has power over the addict. Paradoxically, coaddicts also fear that their efforts will not be enough to eliminate the addiction. When the addicts fail to change, coaddicts interpret that to mean they must try harder. However, since the addicts are in fact powerless, the coaddicts' efforts are doomed to failure. Yet coaddicts allow themselves to believe they have found the right solution. Hope alternates with despair in the coaddicts' lives.

With the addict at the center of the coaddict's world, the

coaddict's life becomes *unmanageable*. Coaddicts report all types of consequences:

- neglect of spiritual life
- loss of friendships
- unusual dreams
- changes in eating and sleeping patterns
- accidents, illnesses, or injury due to the stress of addiction
- loss of time on the job
- decreased ability to work or function
- conflicts with value system or personal ethics
- suicide attempts or thoughts
- financial problems
- takeover of addict's duties and responsibilities
- overextension and overinvolvement in work or outside activities
- self-defeating or degrading behavior

The Coaddict's Checklist on pages 130 and 131 is provided to help spouses, family members, and others identify their coaddictive behaviors.

Once the family has entered the unmanageable double life of the addict, the whole family unit becomes progressively more *isolated*. Participation in the secrecy, enabling, controlling, grandiosity—all generate a collective complicity in the addiction. At a fundamental level, family members understand that and erect *external barriers* to public scrutiny. These barriers also reduce the chances for effective help.

The general family isolation amplifies the loneliness of each of the members. *Increasing distance between family members* becomes the norm in the family. Rather than admitting to a personal need, it is easier for an individual member to be critical of others. When there is a chance for real intimacy, it is

The following are typical coaddictive traits. Simply check off the ones that apply to you. The more items you check, the more you will see a coaddictive pattern in your life. A further step is to record in a private

☐   concealing behavior of the addict

☐   protecting the addict from consequences of behavior

☐   denial of the obvious

☐   alibis, excuses, and justifications to others

☐   feelings of responsibility for the addict's behavior

☐   self-righteous criticism and judgment of the addict

☐   efforts to confront the addict with his or her "problem"

☐   feelings of superiority to the addict

☐   overlooking the addict's behavior

☐   distrust of others outside the family because of the addict

☐   rationalizing the addict's behavior

☐   fantasizing and obsession about the addict's problem

☐   belief that if the addict changed, all problems would disappear

☐   efforts to threaten or exact promises from the addict

☐   strategies to control sexual activity of the addict

☐   attempts to "catch" or trap the addict

☐   being sexual with the addict to prevent the addict from being sexual with others

☐   intense mood swings from high to low

☐   ongoing list of resentments and disappointments

☐   feelings of depression and remorse

☐   loss of friendships

Figure 5.2

CHECKLIST

journal or notebook as many examples as you can remember for each item checked. The result will be a descriptive picture of your total coaddictive system.

- ☐ deterioration of family "pride"
- ☐ secret pacts with other family members
- ☐ feeling distant from other family members
- ☐ distrust of each other within the family
- ☐ loss of self-esteem or self-respect
- ☐ growing self-doubt and fear
- ☐ feeling unique
- ☐ neglect of spiritual pursuits, including prayer or meditation
- ☐ unusual dreams
- ☐ changes in eating or sleeping patterns
- ☐ accidents, illnesses, or injury due to the stress of addiction
- ☐ loss of time on the job
- ☐ decreased ability to work or function
- ☐ suicide attempts or thoughts
- ☐ efforts to control family expenditures, with increasing failure to do so
- ☐ increasing financial problems
- ☐ takeover of the duties and responsibilities of the addict in an effort to keep family life "normal"
- ☐ overextension and overinvolvement in work or outside activities
- ☐ engaging in self-defeating or degrading behavior

evaded by silence or by fighting. Some families stay connected through their fights, but the individual members remain lonely. Because family members do not have *effective linkages* with each other or with outsiders, they make *ineffective responses* to crises. Problems often require everyone's cooperation to solve. Outside help can be necessary, too. Problems that are not resolved—finances, work, parenting—simply add to the unmanageability and personal chaos.

Unmanageability causes family members to feel shameful about their family, although they are quick to defend it. In effect, they have a low concept of themselves as a family and as individuals. Deteriorating family and personal pride validates the core beliefs of each family member who supports the addiction. To understand that connection more fully, one must see the role core beliefs play in the coaddict's world.

THE COADDICT'S CORE BELIEFS

When Joanne's daughter told her she'd been a victim of incest, Joanne did not believe her. In fact, she berated her daughter for even talking like that about her father. Two years later, when her daughter ran away, Joanne learned the truth. She saw that she had enabled her husband's addiction to last two years longer. During treatment she realized that her denial and enabling originated in the whole family's low self-esteem. She wrote in her treatment autobiography:

> And I've come to find out that our whole family was sick and needed help. The help that I started to get for my husband and daughter ended up being for me, too. And I've learned a lot and I've come a long way. Self-esteem seems to be very low in all of these families,

including mine. I guess as a child I just wasn't given the love that I needed. I don't know if that reflects on my parents any. Maybe they just didn't know how to give it either. I think that's why incest remains in the family from generation to generation, and it's commonly called the family secret. No one talks about it, no one lets on. Parents don't want to admit that they might be bad parents or have something wrong with them.

Coaddicts operate with the belief "I am basically a bad, unworthy person." Because they share this belief with the addicts, they participate in the addictive system easily. Coaddicts grow up in families in which their self-worth is constantly in jeopardy. Feelings of inadequacy and failure parallel the addicts' sense of unworthiness. Not believing there are any options, coaddicts tolerate abusive, humiliating, and degrading behavior. Being with an addict furthers the myth of "unlovability."

Self-righteous disdain often masks the interior fears of the coaddict. Also, aggressive and critical controlling behavior switches with compliant, enabling roles. Coaddicts report that these switches can occur within moments of each other. Either position shares a martyrdom role, in which the coaddict is being "victimized."

Joanne described how these roles worked in her family:

I have come to realize that I sometimes take the place of my daughter and she becomes the wife and mother. I start acting just like a little girl. No wonder incest occurred so easily. I have also come to realize that my husband sometimes expects me to act like his mother, okaying things he does and even telling him what to do and still he tells me that if I am ever like his mom he will leave me. Insane? You bet.

The beliefs and impaired thinking of the addict "fit" well with the controlling or enabling behavior of the coaddict. Reacting to judgment and criticism as deserved, addicts also use it to justify abusive and compulsive behavior. When co-addicts are submissive and compliant, addicts feel burdened, critical, and exploited. Being responsible for all the family's decision making, for example, may make the addict into a "parent" for the coaddict, as opposed to a partner. These feelings also serve as a rationale for addictive behavior.

Coaddicts add to their first belief a second: "No one would love me as I am." Coaddicts in relationships reflect their basic distrust of other people. To be in a relationship engages the three coaddictive fears: that coaddicts would lose their identities in the relationship, that they would be forced to deny what they know is real, and that fulfilling their needs would have a price. To tell others the painful "secrets" would guarantee abandonment. To be honest with or vulnerable to the addict would sacrifice the safety of being self-righteous or compliant. Coaddicts, like the addicts, assume that they are responsible for all the pain in loved ones.

Joanne wrote about how she kept her distance:

> I have really built up an indifferent attitude toward my husband, and by doing this I have somehow managed to put a wall of mistrust around me. This has kept me from experiencing the warmth of others. If someone hurt me I laughed rather than cried. I didn't want them to know I was in pain. I can't ever remember being held as a child even though I wanted to be. I still do. I would shrug off an arm that was put around me and wouldn't let anyone hold my hand for fear I would get too close to them. I remember the first time my counselor put her arm around me. I just broke down in tears that I had

never had before and sank into her arms. I needed someone to hold me and understand my pain. I didn't have to be anyone special or anything for her to care, and because of that I am learning to care and share my love. I can reach out to another and tell them I understand more easily every day. I wouldn't have done that six months ago even if I felt like it. *Love doesn't have a price tag*, and as I experience the hope this program gives me and accept myself, I am becoming able to love others and I am finding I have a lot to give back, and trust seems to be there, too. I have reached out and learned that not everyone goes away. Some reach back, and we get a lot of support from each other.

Coaddicts go to extreme lengths to appear self-sufficient. They appear unaffected by any problems and will expend intense energy to conceal problems. In fact, coaddicts will take on many extra responsibilities, being all things to all people. They often seek relationships in which they dominate or nurture because they can be intimate with minimum risk. Just as coaddicts sometimes make addicts into "parents," coaddicts will treat addicts as "another child in the family." This self-sufficient exterior protects the secrets of the family and precludes the coaddict from having to acknowledge his or her personal needs. Also, the internal belief that the coaddict is responsible for everything is acted out.

Joanne's overly responsible behavior was typical:

My husband used to bring me home his paycheck every week. He was a very good husband. And I took care of paying all the bills out of it. But he wanted some spending money. I never could tell him that there wasn't enough money to go around and I didn't have enough to give him spending money, so I gave him what he

wanted and robbed Peter to pay Paul and eventually
Peter and Paul wanted to be paid. And then I'd have to
hide the bills. I would even hide things that I bought for
me. After all, didn't his paycheck come totally to me?
He could have gone out and spent it on something else,
but he always brought it home to me. Somehow I
should have the power to make it stretch. I finally had
to admit that I had limitations. And the phone calls
from the collectors sure proved unmanageability. I
learned about that in part of the First Step, too. I came to
realize that I'm not responsible for my husband and his
actions. Many times I made excuses for the things he
said or did that I somehow didn't agree with, and I felt
others didn't agree with, either. I'd try to explain away
his reasoning. I've learned that my first obligation is to
manage my own life. Let go of what I can't control and
trust God to help me. It's a daily thing and can only be
done one day at a time.

Addicts often rely on coaddicts to pick up the pieces, especially as powerlessness and unmanageability increase.
However, addicts may start to be critical of coaddicts' efforts,
criticizing mistakes they've made while performing extra
chores. For instance, if the wife has taken over the family's
bookkeeping, her husband may fault her if the checkbook
doesn't balance. The criticism stems from the addicts feeling
progressively more useless and without a place in the coaddicts' lives. The addicts feel unneeded, especially when the
coaddicts are busy nurturing others, like children. The coaddicts' involvements serve as further justification for compulsiveness.

The next core belief also parallels the addict's belief: "My
needs are never going to be met if I have to depend upon

others." The coaddict's desperate need for love and nurturing exceeds any one person's ability to respond. The coaddict's high expectations fit with other efforts to control the addict. When he or she is disappointed because the addict failed to meet the highest expectations, the coaddict's rage becomes internalized, resulting in despair, self-pity, and resentment. These down times alternate with periodic exhilaration and hope that things will change. Conniving manipulation and criticism are based on the assumption that if the addict were to meet the high standards, the coaddict's needs would be met. The addict becomes the source of the coaddict's self-worth and good feelings. The conviction that the coaddict will have to pay for love and care pervades all relationships. To be loved and cared for with no requirements goes beyond the coaddict's experience.

Joanne aptly described this process:

> My ability to respond to my needs and to the needs of others is really hard. Most of the time I simply react. I often try to be responsible for everyone and everything. When that happens it results in a lot of frustration and a lot of anger, even self-pity. I have had to realize that I am only responsible for me and my reactions and try real hard to quit controlling. At first I was trying to blame my husband or anyone else who was available for what was going on and what I was going through. I had to learn that I alone had to be responsible for my faults. I had to stop nagging, complaining, and criticizing. I had to stop being the manager, accuser, and judge, and I had to stop forcing issues. Forcing issues came easy and still does. It is hard to let go.

Martyrdom is a part of the coaddicts' systematic efforts to make themselves indispensable to the addicts. In exchange, the coaddicts expect the addicts to furnish proof of care and love. Failure to do so results in further efforts to reform or shape up the addicts or in self-righteous punishment and rejection. The coaddicts do not communicate personal needs, only disappointed expectations. Preoccupation with the addicts often results in the denial or tolerance of the addicts' behavior. Coaddicts "keep score" of what is owed in the relationship. The more coaddicts do for the addicts, the more they expect from them.

Addicts fail to perceive coaddicts' needs. Partially, their failure stems from the addictive preoccupation and sexualization of all needs. The coaddict's behavior, however, also obscures the issues in the relationship. The addict grows resentful of the expectations yet also feels a sense of failure for not meeting them—which no one person could do. Coaddictive judgments simply document what addicts already fear to be true. Yet, addicts remain confident that coaddicts will not leave their relationship because of the coaddictive preoccupation. As long as they are still judging, they are still there.

The final core belief is the only one in which coaddicts differ substantially from addicts. Instead of seeing sex as the most important need, coaddicts often believe, "Sex is the most important sign of love." As children, coaddicts confused sexual interest with care. They were just as lonely, but they learned quickly that they could gain attention, warmth, and care by acting cute and sexy. Also, the uglier someone feels, whether truly so or not, the more sexual he or she acts to gain the attention needed.

Sex also became a vehicle by which fundamental nurturing needs were met. If a child was sexually abused by someone important to him or her, that further confirmed the belief. Being sexually abused teaches the child that in order to have a relationship, one has to be sexual. Abuse victims grow up as adults who believe that sex is the price to be paid for nurturing. If one of these children eventually marries a person whose major source of comfort is sex, their relationship relies on sexual intensity to carry it.

Therefore, coaddicts have the conviction that sexual attention affirms the whole person. Sex becomes one of the most tangible trade-offs for love. Therefore, coaddicts have a great fear of being unattractive and sexually inadequate. When the addicts are sexual with others, the coaddicts feel total personal rejection. Given the stakes, coaddicts have difficulty exploring or enjoying their own sexuality. Because of the repeated disappointments in sex as a way to meet relationship needs, they continue to distrust. Experiences where the coaddicts are exploited foster deep resentment and rage, which further validate all the coaddictive core beliefs.

Both men and women coaddicts have been reported posing as another person in a chat room and "having an affair with their own spouse" as a way to gain the partner's attention. Yet they betray themselves as well. Others say they would put their partners under various forms of surveillance, including hiring private detectives and installing software to track their activities, and would be sexual in exchange for love. Coaddicts may find themselves being sexual when they do not wish to be or, worse, participating in sexual behavior that is degrading or humiliating. Coaddicts may also dress or act seductively to get attention. Efforts to control the addict's sexual obsession include the use of sex to prevent the addict from being sexual with others. Sexual attitudes of the coaddicts may reflect their other external themes of indifference, self-sufficiency, self-righteousness, and martyrdom.

Addicts feel confused by the conflicting signals from the coaddicts about sex. Often addicts misinterpret the coaddicts' needs for relationships as sexual overtures. As a result, addicts totally fail to understand the exploited feelings of the coaddicts. The addicts feel ashamed when sexual feelings are not returned, since that confirms that their sexual intensity is bad. Also, addicts resent the coaddicts' efforts to control and judge their sexual behavior, all of which perpetuates their addiction system. The core beliefs of coaddicts are summarized in The World of the Coaddict, which appears on pages 142 thorugh 145.

THE FAMILY ILLNESS

The delicate balance of human ecology we call a family relies on the interdependence of its members. When issues around self-esteem, relationships, and needs are not resolved, the impact is felt throughout the entire web of relationships. When those issues evolve into addiction and coaddiction, the loving bonds become a prison. The entire family—maybe for generations—participates in thought and action.

Understandably, addiction of all kinds thrives in such an environment. Alcoholism and compulsive overeating are frequent partners in the sexual addiction dance. The husband justifies his sexual addiction because "she is always drunk." The wife who gains 150 pounds as an expression of her rage or as a statement about sexuality is also doing something her husband cannot control. Sometimes both partners act out sexually and become codependent with each other. In a family with *multiple addictions*, the varieties of addiction and coaddiction simply reinforce one another. Each addiction may involve different behaviors, but shares a common addiction system.

When the family balance is upset by the addiction of one or more members, the task of renewal requires that each member—addict or coaddict, child or grandparent—takes responsibility for his or her part. The shift of the energy from blaming others to ownership of personal action creates a new environment of trust. Taking responsibility starts with a thorough knowledge of one's own belief system. That is the goal of the next chapter.

CORE BELIEF 1
SELF-IMAGE: I am basically a bad,
              unworthy person.

Interior World

Coaddicts grow up in families in which their self-worth is in constant jeopardy. Feelings of inadequacy and failure parallel the addicts' sense of unworthiness. Not believing there are any options, coaddicts tolerate abusive, humiliating, and degrading behavior. Coaddicts are obsessed with sex since sex is the proof of love.

Exterior World

Self-righteous contempt often masks the coaddict's interior fears. Aggressive, critical, controlling behavior switches with compliance and enabling. Either position shares a martyrdom role in which the coaddict is being "victimized."

Addicts'
Response to
Coaddicts

Addicts are in a self-serving double bind in the relationship. When coaddicts are critical and judgmental, addicts use this to justify abusive, compulsive behavior. When coaddicts are submissive and compliant, addicts feel burdened, exploited, and critical. These feelings also serve as a rationale for addictive behavior.

Figure 5.3

COADDICT

CORE BELIEF 2
RELATIONSHIPS: No one would love me
as I am.

Interior World

Coaddicts in relationships reflect their basic distrust of others' love and care for them. To be in a relationship engages the three coaddictive fears: that coaddicts would lose their identities in the relationship, that they would be forced to deny what they know to be true, and that meeting their needs would have a price. To tell others the painful "secrets" would guarantee abandonment. To be honest with the addicts would sacrifice the safety of being self-righteous or compliant. Coaddicts, like addicts, assume that they are responsible for all the pain in loved ones.

Exterior World

Coaddicts go to extreme lengths to appear self-sufficient. They seem unaffected by any problems and will expend intense energy to conceal problems. In fact, they will take on many extra responsibilities, being all things to all people. In general, they often seek relationships in which they can dominate or nurture so they can be intimate with minimum risk. This self-sufficient exterior protects the family secrets. Also, the internal belief that the coaddicts are responsible for everything is acted out.

**Addicts'
Response to
Coaddicts**

Addicts rely on coaddicts to pick up the pieces— especially as powerlessness and unmanageability increase. Yet addicts may start to be critical of coaddicts' efforts when they assume extra responsibility. Internally, addicts start to feel progressively more useless and without places in the coaddicts' lives. Addicts feel unneeded, especially when coaddicts are busy nurturing others, such as children. The coaddicts' involvements serve as further justification for compulsiveness.

CORE BELIEF 3
NEEDS: My needs are never going to be met
if I have to depend upon others.

Interior World

Coaddicts' desperate need for love and nurturing exceeds any one person's ability to respond. They make perfectionistic demands on all aspects of the addicts' behavior in a misdirected attempt to guarantee satisfaction of their needs. When they are disappointed by the addicts' failure to meet the impossible demands, rage becomes internalized, resulting in despair, self-pity, and resentment. These down times alternate with periodic hope and exhilaration that things will change. Coaddicts' conniving manipulation and criticism are based on the assumption that if the addicts met the high standards, needs would be met. Addicts become the coaddicts' source of self-worth and good feelings. The conviction that the coaddicts will have to pay for love and care pervades all relationships. To be affirmed with no requirements goes beyond the coaddicts' experience.

Exterior World

Martyrdom accompanies the coaddicts' systematic efforts to make themselves indispensable. In exchange, coaddicts expect addicts to furnish proof of care and love. Failure to do so results in further efforts to reform the addicts or in self-righteous punishment and rejection. Coaddicts do not communicate personal needs, only disappointment in unmet expectations. Preoccupation with addicts often results in the denial or tolerance of addicts' behavior. Coaddicts "keep score" of what is owed in the relationship. The more coaddicts do for the addicts, the more they expect in return.

Addicts'
Response to
Coaddicts

Addicts fail to perceive coaddicts' needs. Partially, their failure stems from the addictive preoccupation and sexualization of all needs. The coaddicts' behavior, however, also obscures the issues in the relationship. Addicts grow resentful of the coaddicts' expectations, yet also feel a sense of failure for not meeting them—which no one person could do. Coaddictive judgments simply document what addicts already fear to be true. Yet addicts remain assured that coaddicts will not leave while they are coaddictively preoccupied—as long as they are still judging, they are still there.

Figure 5.3 *(Continued)*

CORE BELIEF 4
SEXUALITY: Sex is the most important
sign of love.

Interior World

Coaddicts believe sexual attention proves they are lovable. Sex becomes a trade-off for love. Therefore, coaddicts have a great fear of being unattractive and sexually inadequate. When addicts are sexual with others, coaddicts feel total personal rejection, adding to their sense of unlovability. Given the stakes, coaddicts have difficulty exploring or enjoying their own sexuality. Exploitive experiences foster deep resentment and rage, which further validate all the coaddictive core beliefs.

Exterior World

Because sex is a trade-off for love, coaddicts may find themselves being sexual when they do not wish to be or, worse, participating in sexual behavior that is degrading and humiliating. Coaddicts may also dress or act seductively to get attention. Efforts to control the addicts' sexual obsession include the use of sex to manipulate addicts to prevent them from being sexual with others. Sexual attitudes of the coaddicts can continue the external themes of self-sufficiency, self-righteousness, and martyrdom.

Addicts'
Response to
Coaddicts

Addicts feel confused by the coaddicts' contradictory signals about sex. Often addicts misinterpret the coaddicts' need for relationship as sexual overtures and then totally fail to understand the coaddicts' feelings of being exploited. Addicts are ashamed when sexual feelings are not returned, since that confirms that their sexual intensity is bad. Also, there are feelings of resentment about the coaddicts' efforts to control and judge the addicts' sexual behavior, all of which perpetuates the addiction cycle of the addicts.

CHAPTER 6

The Belief System

◨ ◨ ◨

> The contradictions which develop between the affectionate
> experiences of a childhood and the dehumanized relation-
> ships of adulthood create insoluble conflicts for both sexes.
> These conflicts take different forms in women and men. . . .
> Our society creates psychic war within the two sexes and so
> perpetuates the war between them.
>
> —Helen Block Lewis, *Psychic War in Men and Women*

The image of the seductive siren so powerful that even the
bravest of men would succumb to her charms is as old as
Ulysses' trek around the Aegean Sea. Powerlessness before
women is a long-standing theme in Western classical and current literature. Part of every man can identify with some of
the cartoon stereotypes: Dagwood being outmaneuvered by
Blondie; Charlie Brown laughed at derisively by Lucy and her
friends; or Hagar the Horrible becoming Hagar the Helpless
in front of his wife. As a theme, male powerlessness is as
much a symptom of the sexual ills of our culture as are the
many examples of the exploitation of women. The male sexual addict most visibly manifests this, for he believes he is
powerless in front of women. This chapter focuses on how
cultural beliefs support the dysfunctional core beliefs of the
addict. The central sexual beliefs of our culture are prime

ingredients in the addictive systems that destroy men and women and their coaddicts.

In the perceptive words of Helen Block Lewis, we live in an exploitative society that "injures the two sexes differently."[1] Lewis characterizes men as "expendable warriors" who, in their dominant role of providers, must relinquish the human bonding that nourishes every human soul. Women, "the inferior childbearers," according to Lewis, maintain their capacity to nurture but to a significant degree give up their self-determination. Men become economic symbols. Women become sex symbols. The quintessential expression of the transaction is prostitution, that is, money for sex. Its most injurious form is rape. From an addiction perspective, cultural expectations contribute to the addiction for both men and women.

Lewis points to societies in which providing and relationship responsibilities are shared. Responsibility for sexual initiation is also mutual. Either man or woman can reach out for one another without fear. Sexuality becomes an open and loving expression of the affection bond. When both men and women feel powerless in the presence of the other, sexuality can become a diminishing experience. Combining these cultural perceptions with the core beliefs of the addict generates compulsivity of enormous power.

THE CULTURAL BELIEFS

Warren Farrell, author of *The Liberated Man*, suggests that we are socializing or training men to be minirapists and women to be minimasochists. We develop in men the psychological characteristics of a rapist, but within an acceptable structure. The key factor in this socialization is that men are given the responsibility to initiate relationships and women are trained to be overcome. Farrell writes:

What is the effect on women of men's role to do the overcoming? Men learn to protect themselves from the hurt of rejection by turning women into sex objects. It is easier to accept rejection by an object than by a human being. If we can turn women into objects and sex into a game, talking about how far we got and whether we scored, it helps us avoid looking at why we were rejected. It helps us gain the courage to try even harder the next time (as we would in fulfilling an athletic role . . .). Each time a woman does not share in the initiative of obtaining the type of sexual involvement she wants, she is contributing to the use of herself as a sex object. Each time a man gives a woman negative feedback when she takes the initiative, he is contributing to his own frustration, to his anger and contempt for women (as objects that need to be persuaded to enjoy themselves), and to his need to use a woman as a sex object to protect himself from the very vulnerability he is reinforcing. Many women complain about men not being in touch with their feelings. It is dysfunctional for a man to be in touch with his feelings if he is going to be opening himself up to experiencing the pain of rejection. It is even more dysfunctional if he has to recover from the rejection and try again.[2]

Let us use men as an example. We will focus on women addicts later in the chapter. If a man comes from a family in which he feels bad about himself, has little confidence that women would want to be with him, and believes that sex is the one comfort he cannot do without, addiction can occur. Place that same man in a culture that makes women into sexual objects, and addiction will thrive. The belief system, the impaired thinking, the preoccupation and obsession, and the ritualization are all enhanced by cultural perceptions. People overlook powerlessness because it is the nature of men "to be carried away." As long as we depersonalize sex, men do not have to be responsible.

Addicts often talk about the difficulty of recovery. They live in a culture in which advertising efforts portray sex as central to the good life. Addicts already struggle with personal obsession. They have to struggle with cultural sexual obsession, as well. If the male addict shared with men friends his wish to stop having affairs or seeing prostitutes, his friends might well respond, "Why would you want to do that?" Part of the male image is the conquest of women. Another part of the image, which advertising people know, is that men are susceptible to sexual overtures. They are perceived as powerless when it comes to their sexual needs. They will do what they can "to get it," and the best man is the one who succeeds in doing just that.

Given the pervasive quality of these attitudes, they have a severe impact on the addicts' core beliefs. The chart The Male Sexual Addict's Beliefs about Sex, Men, and Women," pages 152 and 153, summarizes common perceptions held by male sexual addicts. These perceptions result from the fusion of faulty core beliefs with dysfunctional cultural attitudes. The perceptions reflect the addicts' low self-worth and alienation and their basic confusion that sexual expression will relieve their personal pain. Also reflected are the conflicting cultural roles of men and women. Stated in its most extreme form of dysfunction, women decide whether men will have sex or not. Men control economic security.

For the addict, two themes emerge. The first is an overwhelming need for sexual contact. He experiences this need in an environment that bombards him with sexual titillation from newsstands, the Internet, television, and advertising campaigns that use sex to promote products. The second is a profound hopelessness, believing as he does that his sexual needs will not be met by other people. Or if they are partially met, it will not be enough. Seduction, illicit behavior, and manipulation all become options and also add excitement to the addictive cycle. For some addicts the ultimate bind emerges when they believe they must have it, but no one will give it to them. That profound sense of powerlessness can escalate to the use of force and the victimization of others.

An important connection exists between powerlessness and victimization. Rollo May's already classic description of this relationship in *Power and Innocence* shows that in a very real sense it generates "madness." A person who feels powerless to influence his or her situation is extremely angry or mad. The more powerless the person feels, the more prone that person is to violence. May suggests that this is a helpful way to understand the anger characteristic of insanity or "madness."[3]

The levels of addiction described in chapter 2 provide a framework for understanding how the sexual addict's victimization of others is connected to his powerlessness. The more he believes he cannot influence his relationships with women, the more likely he is to perform Level Two and Three behaviors. Built on the premise that he is powerless, the addict's belief system becomes an elaborate structure of myths and delusions that he sees as reality but that in fact

- diminish his self-worth
- limit his possibilities in relationships
- justify his victimization in terms of his needs
- connect sexuality with survival

THE MALE SEXUAL ADDICT'S BELIEFS

THE CORE BELIEFS	THE ADDICT'S SELF-PERCEPTION
1. Self-image: I am basically a bad, unworthy person.	I am not attractive, personally or physically. A woman would not choose me.
2. Relationships: No one would love me as I am.	I will have to convince a woman to be with me.
3. Needs: My needs are never going to be met if I have to depend upon others.	My needs can only be met by luck or chance, careful strategizing, or the accumulation of money or power.
4. Sexuality: Sex is my most important need.	I need sex all the time, cannot get enough, and must not pass up any opportunities. I am the only one who needs sex this much.

Figure 6.1

ABOUT SEX, MEN, AND WOMEN

THE ADDICT'S PERCEPTION OF MEN

Other men are more attractive, more successful, and more likely to be chosen by women.

Men have to initiate relationships. Other men are more effective than I.

Men have external power in jobs and money but will give in on issues to keep women happy.

Men are more sexual than women and more free to enjoy it. They will take sex whenever they can get it and cannot be trusted around women.

THE ADDICT'S PERCEPTION OF WOMEN

Women choose men who are not like me. They prefer stronger, smarter, and more successful men.

Women can wait, pick, and choose to accept relationship offers.

Women make decisions at home and in other areas. They are impressed by money, possessions, and security.

Women are less sexual than men and have to be coaxed into being sexual. Consequently, they are responsible for moral behaviors and can use sex as a reward or punishment.

The more dysfunctional the belief system, the higher the probability that the addict's pattern of sexual compulsiveness will include the types of victimization found in Levels Two and Three.

All addicts must alter their fundamental "core beliefs" in order to recover. In that sense, they are no different from anyone confronted with personal problems. A good example is the pioneering publication *The Structure of Magic*, by Richard Bandler and John Grinder.[4] By examining the work of a number of successful therapists from different schools of thought, they distilled an important commonality: the most effective therapists were those who were able to help their clients broaden their perceptions of possible choices. In other words, most people have problems because they believe that there are only certain options—usually self-defeating—open to them. The therapist must assist them in discovering new possibilities for themselves and others. Bandler and Grinder describe this task as basically a problem of language and conception—that there are more options than the patient believed there were.

Recovery means seeking new options, not only for the addict but also for the entire family. Family members have faulty beliefs—both cultural and core beliefs—as part of their co-addiction. Together the whole family can take on the search for alternate ways of being together.

THE FAMILY BELIEFS

The families filed into the room with an easiness that belied the fact that up until a few weeks ago they had never met. Children scampered. Adults chatted. For all intents and purposes, it could have been a church meeting. What these families shared, however, was sexual addiction. At least one member of each family was sexually compulsive to an extent that there were serious consequences and the family was referred to treatment.

In this treatment program, 70 percent of the families also had a chemically dependent member. Weight was also an issue for many. An inordinate number of wives, for example, had intestinal bypass surgery. The desperation and eagerness of the families to learn was reflected in the silence and quick attention the instructor received as she gathered them together.

The session started with the instructor explaining that in order to understand addiction, one needed to explore the belief system that gives it life. A belief system, she explained, contains an elaborate set of rules, values, and myths created by the family and culture and integrated into the family. All behavior and options are judged by these beliefs. A set of judgments about oneself (core beliefs) exists within that belief system, such as one's own sexuality. These judgments are key to the addictive process for all family members.

The instructor asked the families to divide into separate groups—adult men, adult women, adolescent boys, adolescent girls, and children. Each group received sheets of newsprint and marking pens. Each group appointed a secretary. The instructor then gave the assignment: What do you believe to be true about sex, power in the family, attractiveness, and money? The instructor asked the secretary to record these beliefs. The children were given a special instruction: What have you heard in your home about sex and what have you heard about money?

Within the men's group, the discussion started with a joke that was followed by nervous laughter, a signal of their anxiety. Slowly and then with greater enthusiasm the ideas started to flow onto the page:

Men have to initiate sex.
Men need it more than women.
Men have to pay for it.
Every man will try to get sex if he can.
Men are attracted to women; women aren't attracted to
    men.
Women don't need it—can do without sex.
Women have to be warmed up.
Women's sexual interest declines after marriage.
Women decide whether to have sex or not.
Women tease—keep you guessing.
Men will chase it—give up more to get it.
Women use it as a weapon or reward.
Men are responsible for earning money, women for spend-
    ing it.

As the men talked, they realized that they had a number of beliefs in common. Women were seen as determining whether men will have what they "desperately" want—sex. They felt anger about women who "tease," about times when women abandon men, and about the power women have over men. They commonly acknowledged how they fear they have "missed out" on sexual experience. They shared resentment about being only as good as their jobs or their income. As a group they believed they could easily be replaced, as long as the money kept coming.

Meanwhile, the women also compiled their list, as angry and untrusting as the men's list:

Men treat women as objects.
Men have "their brains in their pants."
Men cannot be intimate or close—too masculine for that!
Men are not trustworthy.
Men use their economic power—will not share it.

Women are "less" if they are honest about how sexual they feel.

Women suffer a double standard.

Women control with sex.

Women have to raise families "alone."

Women have to be "thin."

The tenor of the women's conversation also sounded angry, as well as punctuated with jokes to relieve the tension. One woman talked of how she hated being something to drain her husband's body so he could sleep. Others quietly nodded their heads in assent. Another added how she used sex to reward or affirm, but not to enjoy. She talked further about her deep self-doubts as to her sexual adequacy. Yet another talked of feeling "trapped"—being unable to leave her marriage. She constantly increased her tolerance to things she hated because she was afraid of being alone and with no means of support.

The instructor then asked each group to have a representative read each list and explain the listings. The men started. As they finished, the instructor asked the women how they would feel if they believed that each of the responses by the men were true—not necessarily that they were, but if they *believed* they were. The women acknowledged that they would feel full of rage.

They were particularly struck by the theme of how the men perceived women as in charge of their sexual relationships.

A spirited discussion started about what the men meant by teasing. The instructor intervened, pointing out that they needed to continue. When the women presented their list, the instructor asked the men for their reactions. Initially, the men kept silent. Then one man shared two reactions. The first was that he could see why the couples fought so much. The second was that it was helpful for him to realize that everybody was experiencing the same things.

Then the instructor asked the adolescents to present their lists. The lists were parallel to the adults' lists. Teenage boys talked about the paralyzing fear of rejection and the pressure to impress. Girls talked of the helplessness of waiting to be picked and of the efforts to gain attention without being obvious.

Next the instructor turned to the children and had them share what they had heard about these issues in their homes. The halting presentation of the younger children provided a painful perspective for everyone. Phrases like "you were a whore" (dad to mom) or "you're not old enough to know about that" (parent to child) brought glistening tears to parents' eyes. The overwhelming expression of sadness and loneliness was incredibly poignant as the adults recognized that what their own children were experiencing now was but an echo of their own early years.

The instructor asked the parents to share with the group memories they had of their own childhoods. One mother spoke of how frightened she was when her dad was sexual with her when she was twelve and how she thought his attraction for her was her fault. A father spoke about how harshly he was disciplined for masturbating. Another shared how as a kid he believed that his parents were not sexual and that only he had those feelings, which were bad to have. He felt he had to pretend he was not sexual in order to be in his family. A woman talked of how from early on in life she was aware that being sexual was a way for her to have her needs met. Simply put, sex was the price one paid.

The instructor then elaborated on the emerging concept that beliefs about sexuality are often recreated with each generation. When negative messages about sexuality join with distorted cultural expectations of men and women, intimacy becomes warped and communications become limited. In fact, the secrecy and shame connected with sexual behavior make it more difficult to get accurate information to dispel myths that might be hurtful. Here again is an environment in which sexual addiction can thrive.

The instructor used the example of the shared belief that "men were not trustworthy" when it came to sex. For the addict, the belief that men in general are not trustworthy fosters impaired thinking like "I am only doing what everyone else is." Essentially, the belief justifies his obsession. For the coaddict who sees her husband as another "untrustworthy" man, she concludes that she has to go to some extraordinary effort to control his behavior. Her impaired thinking tells her that she is responsible for what he does. She becomes preoccupied with the addict's behavior.

The instructor suggested that an alternative exists for both of them. Understanding that both men and women are fundamentally intensely sexual alters the view of the world of the addict and coaddict alike. Each has to take responsibility for his or her own sexual feelings. Addicts no longer need to feel compelled to insane behavior in order to meet their needs. Coaddicts can focus their energy on developing their own sexuality as opposed to being obsessed with the sexuality of the addict. Sharing sexual initiative as well as economic opportunity can displace feelings of jeopardy and exploitation. When both addicts and coaddicts can accept their sexuality as an exciting and rich part of relationships, old myths that equate sexual feelings with being bad are dispelled. By challenging beliefs and cultural expectations, family members can find a path out of addiction.

With that as her final point, the instructor brought the evening to a close. They all made a large circle in which they shared reflections about what they had learned that evening.

As the group broke up, there was much joking and teasing as the families said good-bye.

Treatment programs for sexual addiction offer educational workshops for the addicts and their families, like the one just described, to help families understand the various facets of beliefs and family life that are part of the addiction. In fact, many programs use a combination of education and therapy to dismantle those operational beliefs which support the addiction, as well as to supply new tools and options. By far the toughest task that therapists face when working with families is helping all the members of the family acknowledge their own faulty beliefs. Each member turns family and cultural beliefs into statements about who he or she is. "A bad man is oversexed" becomes "I am a bad man because of my sexual feelings." These self-judgments form the basic elements of a self-concept. They are the "core beliefs."

THE CORE BELIEFS

In the 1977 movie *Looking for Mr. Goodbar*, Diane Keaton ably plays Theresa, a young woman who entered the double life of the sexual addict. In her external world she was known as a compassionate and generous teacher of deaf children. She also had a secret life dominated by compulsive sex. Starting with an affair with her college professor, she initiated a series of exploitive and abusive relationships. These progressed to one-night stands and anonymous sex, including ritualistic cruising at bars. The movie ends with Theresa being killed by a sexual partner she had known only a few hours.

The brutality of the ending underlined the movie's powerful statement about the despair of the addict. The scenes of her work as a teacher served as the perfect counterpoint to the underlying drama of her life—in fact, capturing the duality of which addicts often speak. The story of Theresa helps to illustrate the connections between family, cultural, and core beliefs. Since Theresa is a woman addict, the cultural expectations are reversed, revealing the belief dynamics more clearly. In fact, Theresa's experience points out the role that beliefs play in the whole addictive system.

Theresa comes from a rigid, Catholic family with proscriptive attitudes about sexuality. For example, at one point in the movie, Theresa's encounter with a nun on the street reminds her of the negative messages of her upbringing. Theresa is not alone in her family in struggling with compulsive sexual behavior or the proscriptive rules of the family. Her sister is constantly at odds with her parents. The sister becomes pregnant and is unable to determine who the father is. She agrees to marry a man she has known for four hours. Their marriage has a steady diet of group sex and porn movies. Theresa is repelled and attracted at the same time.

With a dominating alcoholic father, spontaneity and intimacy were extremely limited in Theresa's family. Worse, Theresa had a dramatic bout with polio at age eleven. While there was some physical deformity, the emotional scars were deeper. Her disfigured back became a symbol throughout the movie of her feelings of being unacceptable and unworthy as a person—her core beliefs.

Unworthiness as a person was the cornerstone of Theresa's belief system. She rejected men who initiated sincere relationships because of her fear and distrust. She opted instead for a freewheeling sexuality that precluded lasting relationships. Sexual obsession took over her life. The title, *Looking for Mr. Goodbar*, really referred to a search for intimacy and nurturing. Theresa's core beliefs precluded normal relationship possibilities and held sexuality as the only trustable human exchange with one exception: Theresa trusted the deaf kids because they needed her. In that sense her story parallels so many addicts who are in helping professions—physicians, ministers, teachers, therapists, nurses, and social workers. One way these people can trust relationships in their external world is when they are clearly needed.

Impaired thinking for Theresa stemmed from her belief system. For example, she complained to some of her sex partners about her resentment of men who tried to pay her for sex. Her anger betrayed how removed she was from the reality of how degrading her sexual experiences were. Her beliefs that she was not worthwhile and that sex would meet her needs obscured reality, including her eroding sense of self-respect.

Theresa, like all addicts, made attempts to stop her compulsive addictive cycle. She spoke of her "last night" of cruising in an effort to stop, which failed. The futility of her efforts was most poignant in a conversation Theresa had with a bartender. She invited him to have a drink with her. He declined, saying that for him even one drink was too many. Her poignant reply was, "Yeah, I have that trouble with men."

As her addiction progressed, Theresa became more and more isolated. Like so many addicts, she refused to even sleep with a sex partner after being sexual. The ever-present belief system did not allow for any relationship connection beyond sex. In Theresa's mind, if she let someone sleep with her, he would discover her basic unworthiness and reject her.

The unmanageability of her life increased. Sexual bingeing and heavy drug use caused her to oversleep and come late to school, creating a serious breach with her students, the one group of people to whom she was still close. Her unmanageability and despair confirmed what she believed to be "truths" about her own unworthiness and the undependability of others.

The fundamental paradox of the movie is that the addiction would have been less obvious if the central figure had been a man. By some cultural standards Theresa's behavior would have been less obviously deviant for a man. Part of the movie's success in conveying its theme lies in making the pain of addiction more evident by casting a woman in the role of the addict.

Theresa, as a character, creates a special glimpse into the impact that cultural expectations have on women addicts. The image of the good woman as the guardian of morality who "needs to be overcome" by the right words, the right moment, or the right mood in order to respond sexually presents an immense contrast to the sexually compulsive woman. While cultural beliefs tend to support a male addict's obsession, they contribute to the shame of women addicts who measure themselves by the same social standards. They add to their shame when they feel they must be the "only" woman who acts this way—and it is that sense of uniqueness which is central to the secret world of any addict. Their loneliness represents the special burdens our culture places on women. That Theresa found herself at odds with the cultural expectations of some of her partners, who expected to pay her, was in fact part of the problem.

All addicts and coaddicts, both men and women, face the same task in recovery: understanding their belief systems and finding alternatives. Each person must unravel the contributions of culture and family to his or her core beliefs. To disrupt the addictive system, each person must enter a process that replaces faulty beliefs with healthy ones. Such a process needs to parallel the life-giving dynamics of a healthy family and culture. Therefore, the recovery process must be one that

- builds relationships
- separates the behavior from the person
- establishes clear guidelines for behavior

- promotes learning from mistakes
- relieves shame about past behavior
- allows for amends to be made
- supplies ongoing support and affirmation
- creates a positive sense of self
- acknowledges the human need for help in both men and women
- is a method for checking reality
- is an ongoing exercise in the development of trust
- provides new options for behavior in relationships
- accepts all family members with their strengths and weaknesses

For close to seventy years, members of Alcoholics Anonymous have lived such a process using the Twelve Steps. Starting with the First Step, the program asks its members to make a realistic appraisal of their situation, to admit or acknowledge that they are part of something that is not only destructive but also stronger than they are. It asks them to have faith and trust in the other members of the fellowship and in a Power greater than themselves. In a committed community, addicts can start anew in the full knowledge that there is help. Part of their exploring new options requires a candid statement about what they have done to others. With the human acceptance of that admission, they can then make amends. To recover, addicts accept an invitation to live a discipline, a collected wisdom, a way of life—the Twelve Steps. There is only one ongoing requirement—that they be willing to pass the principles of the program on to others. For in their helping others, they recycle the new learnings, the affirmations, and the human contact. What had been a destructive cycle of illness becomes a life-generating cycle of health. The Twelve Steps as a process for developing new beliefs about oneself is the focus of the next chapter.

CHAPTER 7

Twelve Steps to Recovery

◻ ◻ ◻

A former federal education department employee was sentenced yesterday to nine months in jail despite his pleas to a Virginia judge that he committed three sex-related misdemeanors because he suffers from a mental illness that caused him to be "addicted to sexual gratification."

—*Washington Post*, April 28, 1982

We admitted we were powerless over our sexual addiction—that our lives had become unmanageable.

—The First Step

The government official had much to lose. He had a wife, seven children ranging in age from eighteen to twenty-seven, and a well-paying government post. His career as a nationally recognized educator grew with the publication of three books on sexual liberation and self-awareness—all of which came to an abrupt halt when he was arrested by Arlington detectives on charges of pimping and prostitution. Specifically, he attempted to recruit customers on behalf of the wife of a former State Department official. The newspaper account of his own words reveals his pain:

"My career is totally destroyed; my reputation as a psychologist and educator is ruined." He clenched his fingers as he stood before the judge and apologized for "promoting a life style I know now is a sickness. Money was never my motivation. I would have paid to do what I did and I did pay a lot of money," he said, thanking the detectives who arrested him for "stopping me before my life went further down the drain, if possible."[1]

Further testimony of the impact of sexual addiction came from his wife, who spoke of the pain she had at not being able to "see any way his behavior was going to change."

There are obvious parallels between sexual compulsiveness and addiction to alcohol. Some sexually addicted families go a step further and start to use the proven principles of the Twelve Steps of Alcoholics Anonymous as a way to change their lives.

Though the Twelve Steps were developed by and for alcoholics, it was only a matter of time before they were utilized as a path for those who had other compulsive disorders, and other Twelve Step groups formed: Gamblers Anonymous, Overeaters Anonymous, and Emotions Anonymous. That it has taken so long for a program to emerge for the sexually compulsive is not surprising, given the complexity and intensity of the issues involved—not to mention the shame. A number of groups use the Twelve Steps as the basis for recovery from sexual addiction.

As early as 1975, groups started independently in places like California, Massachusetts, and Minnesota. People who were familiar with the Twelve Steps and Twelve Traditions of Alcoholics Anonymous generated many groups. However, members of other Twelve Step programs such as Overeaters Anonymous also started groups for sexual addiction. While the compulsive behavior may have differed, all shared the common reality of the sexually addictive system and its destructive cycle. The names varied considerably (Sexual Addicts Anonymous, Sex and Love Addicts Anonymous, Sexaholics Anonymous, Sexual Compulsives Anonymous). The groups varied in how they worked and held their meetings. Yet they shared a common program—the Twelve Steps. Using this program, families who have felt high levels of desperation have been able to turn their lives around. The question remains as to how these Steps can help. The goal of this chapter is to show just that—how the Twelve Steps can work for sexual addicts and coaddicts.

Defining sexual addiction as a "pathological relationship to a mood-altering experience" becomes critical to understanding the impact of the Twelve Steps. Chapter 1 described how the sexual addict's obsession replaced all meaningful relationships in the addict's life. Like the alcoholic, the sexual addict's secret life became more important than all that the addict valued, including family, friends, and work. The addiction system—that is, beliefs, impaired thinking, compulsive behavior, and unmanageability—creates its own momentum that isolates the addict further and further. Chapter 2 specified the wide range of compulsive behaviors experienced by addicts, behaviors that contribute to the addicts' alienation. Chapter 3 showed how the Internet vastly expands addictive possibilities. Chapters 4 and 5 showed how the addict's family contributes to and reinforces the addiction. Family members participate in the illness, intensifying the relationship problems. Rooted in the family experience, four core beliefs are central to the deterioration of relationships for both addicts and coaddicts. To summarize, these faulty core beliefs are:

1. I am basically a bad, unworthy person.
2. No one would love me as I am.

3. My needs are never going to be met if I have to depend upon others.
4. Sex is my most important need (addicts), or sex is the most important sign of love (coaddicts).

Cultural beliefs support these core beliefs, creating a belief system integral to the addiction.

TRANSFORMING BELIEFS THROUGH THE TWELVE STEPS

The Twelve Steps can fundamentally interrupt and alter the addictive system. The Steps can restore the capacity for meaningful relationships by developing in addicts and coaddicts new beliefs to replace dysfunctional or faulty beliefs.

Recovering persons who use the Twelve Steps can say to themselves:

1. I am a worthwhile person deserving of pride.
2. I am loved and accepted by people who know me as I am.
3. My needs can be met by others if I let them know what I need.
4. Sex is but one expression of my need and care for others.

Each of the Twelve Steps contributes to the new beliefs. Some Steps, however, are more key to some core beliefs than others. Without losing sight of the interdependence of each Step in the Twelve Step program, the role of key Steps in the change of each core belief can be shown. By examining each core belief separately, the Twelve Step process emerges as a clear path for addicts and coaddicts to have healthy relationships. It will be helpful to refer to the Twelve Steps listed on pages 169 and 170 as you read on.

THE TWELVE STEPS OF ALCOHOLICS ANONYMOUS*

1. We admitted we were powerless over alcohol—that our lives had become unmanageable.

2. Came to believe that a Power greater than ourselves could restore us to sanity.

3. Made a decision to turn our will and our lives over to the care of God *as we understood Him.*

4. Made a searching and fearless moral inventory of ourselves.

5. Admitted to God, to ourselves, and to another human being the exact nature of our wrongs.

6. Were entirely ready to have God remove all these defects of character.

7. Humbly asked Him to remove our shortcomings.

8. Made a list of all persons we had harmed, and became willing to make amends to them all.

9. Made direct amends to such people wherever possible, except when to do so would injure them or others.

10. Continued to take personal inventory and when we were wrong promptly admitted it.

11. Sought through prayer and meditation to improve our conscious contact with God *as we understood Him,* praying only for knowledge of His will for us and the power to carry that out.

12. Having had a spiritual awakening as the result of these steps, we tried to carry this message to alcoholics, and to practice these principles in all our affairs.

*The Twelve Steps of AA are taken from *Alcoholics Anonymous,* 3d ed., published by AA World Services, Inc., New York, N.Y., 59–60. Reprinted with permission of AA World Services, Inc. (See editor's note on copyright page.)

Figure 7.1

THE TWELVE STEPS OF ALCOHOLICS ANONYMOUS ADAPTED FOR SEXUAL ADDICTS*

1. We admitted we were powerless over our sexual addiction— that our lives had become unmanageable.

2. Came to believe that a Power greater than ourselves could restore us to sanity.

3. Made a decision to turn our will and our lives over to the care of God as we understood Him.

4. Made a searching and fearless moral inventory of ourselves.

5. Admitted to God, to ourselves, and to another human being the exact nature of our wrongs.

6. Were entirely ready to have God remove all these defects of character.

7. Humbly asked Him to remove our shortcomings.

8. Made a list of all persons we had harmed, and became willing to make amends to them all.

9. Made direct amends to such people wherever possible, except when to do so would injure them or others.

10. Continued to take personal inventory and when we were wrong promptly admitted it.

11. Sought through prayer and meditation to improve our conscious contact with God as we understood Him, praying only for knowledge of His will for us and the power to carry that out.

12. Having had a spiritual awakening as the result of these steps, we tried to carry this message to others and to practice these principles in all our affairs.

*Adapted from the Twelve Steps of Alcoholics Anonymous with permission of AA World Services, Inc., New York, N.Y.

Figure 7.2

Core Belief One: I am basically a bad, unworthy person.

This belief expresses the self-concept of addicts and coaddicts. A positive sense of self precedes any possibility of closeness or intimacy. Without that fundamental acceptance of self, nurturing and intimacy can be closed out. Addicts who regard themselves as "unworthy" survive in a secret world in which obsession blocks pain and loneliness and in which they are accountable to no one. Only the addicts know the whole truth. Each effort to quit that fails adds to an addict's sense of hopelessness. By keeping their obsessions secret, addicts, as well as family members, maintain an illusionary sense of control and responsibility.

With the First Step, addicts and coaddicts admit their powerlessness and unmanageability. As the admission removes the veil of secrecy, they find that they share a common problem with others. They realize that their addiction—a potent combination of cultural, family, and personal belief systems— was much more powerful than they were. Their isolation guaranteed the failure of their efforts to control. Instead of secrecy and self-control, the addict or coaddict must admit to others the need for help and receive it.

It helps when the admission of powerlessness occurs in the presence of others who have shared the same problem. The admission is less frightening. Being surrounded by recovering people reinforces honesty. Also, their insight helps the addicts with the greatest realization in terms of the first core belief—that they are not bad persons. Rather, they were part of an illness that was destroying their lives.

By declaring the unmanageability of their lives, addicts and coaddicts are forced to recognize the ways they were destroying themselves and others. The First Step starts addicts and coaddicts on the path to reclaiming reality. Fully acknowledging the consequences of the addiction encourages them to commit to a program that can arrest the illness.

Steps Two and Three ask addicts and coaddicts to make an act of faith that they can recover with the help of a Higher Power. Essentially these are spiritual Steps, yet they do not prescribe a religion. Rather, they invite addicts to stop and reflect about what gives their lives meaning and purpose. This reflective process serves as an antidote to feelings of unworthiness. To establish a relationship with God is the first bridge to trusting relationships with others. Ernest Becker put it most succinctly in his Pulitzer Prize–winning book, *The Denial of Death:*

> Perversion has been called a "private religion"—and that it really is, but it testifies to fear and trembling and not to faith. It is an idiosyncratic symbolic protest of control and safety by those who can rely on nothing—neither their own powers nor the shared cultural map for interpersonal action.[2]

The "private religion" of the secret world must give way to Steps Two and Three. Addicts and coaddicts discover that they are not alone, that they are not abandoned and therefore are not bad and unworthy as they learn to trust a Higher Power and the fellowship.

Steps One, Two, and Three combine within the addict or coaddict to internalize a new belief: "I am a worthwhile person deserving of pride." A new sense of pride is born. The power of the secret world is broken. Identity and integrity return. Since there is no longer a need to hide, addicts can become open to each other in the fellowship and accessible to others outside the Twelve Step community.

Core Belief Two: No one would love me as I am.

When addicts or coaddicts conclude that they are basically bad persons and thus do not love themselves, they add the parallel belief that no one else would love them, either. Given this belief, the only path for them is to project an unreal image that protects the secrets of the addiction. Addicts and co-addicts live with constant tension, fearing the truth will be discovered and made public. Rejection and abandonment would follow.

Step Four asks for a moral inventory during which addicts and family members must be brutally honest with themselves. This inventory includes strengths as well as weaknesses. An honest appraisal of strengths helps dismantle the basic convictions about being unworthy and unlovable. Assessing weaknesses helps addicts and coaddicts focus on changes they can make, thereby adding hope. Analyzing strengths and weaknesses together continues the Twelve Step theme of reclaiming reality about behavior, beliefs, and impaired thinking.

Step Five requires the sharing of the Fourth Step inventory with another person. This Step, more than any other, challenges the addicts' and coaddicts' beliefs that if someone really knew everything about them, they would be rejected. In the unconditional acceptance of another human being, a great release of pain often occurs. By being sorry for what they have done, addicts experience reconciliation and forgiveness. Because of the spiritual qualities of that experience, clergy are often sought to hear a Fifth Step.

Later in the program, Steps Eight and Nine demand that addicts make a list of people they have harmed and make amends where possible. Going further than the forgiveness in Step Five, the Twelve Step program teaches that addicts and

coaddicts can make up for what they have done. They need
not feel guilt and shame forever. Amends-making gives them
the opportunity for dignity. They learn that when they make a
mistake, they don't need to retreat into the secret world. In
most cases, people will accept their efforts to right the wrongs
they have done.

Steps Four, Five, Eight, and Nine help addicts and coaddicts tap into their own sources of renewal. They find that
they will not be abandoned, as so many of them were in their
families when they were children. Instead, they come to a
new conclusion about themselves: "I am loved and accepted
by people who know me as I am." Their belief allows them to
take responsibility for their behavior, and their behavior becomes more congruent with their values. They can accept
their mistakes, make amends, and receive forgiveness.
Addicts and coaddicts can become responsive and responsible members of the human community.

Core Belief Three: My needs are never going to be met if I have to depend upon others.

While the first two core beliefs dealt with self-acceptance and
intimacy, the third core belief deals with dependency. Addicts
and coaddicts distrust other people, believing themselves to
be unworthy and unlovable. Therefore they conclude that
they cannot depend on others. The addict asks, "Who would
meet the needs of someone unlovable and unworthy? Who
will care, listen, sympathize, and nurture? Who will take over,
be concerned, act on my behalf, give advice, or share their
lives? Who will help me when I am lonely, hurting, or desperate?" Everyone has those needs and feelings. But the depriva-
tion in the lives of addicts and coaddicts leaves them
convinced that those basic human gifts from healthy relation-

ships will never be given to them. This belief leaves addicts and coaddicts rageful, manipulative, and secretive.

When they admit their need by joining a Twelve Step program, addicts and their family members have their first experience in the care of the fellowship. The program has no conditions or restrictions. Addicts and their families receive affirmation simply through admitting their needs. The care they experience provides a basic experience that allows addicts and coaddicts to trust a Higher Power and the human community to supply the care they need and frees them to discard the old self-destructive behaviors they had used to feel better. When addicts and coaddicts depended on their sexual "connections," they found their lives empty and still unsatisfied. Depending on others does bring the fundamental affirmation of themselves as persons. Almost like children, both the addicts and coaddicts have to be taught, or have to relearn, how to let others know about their needs. As they learn to ask, they discover a new belief: "My needs can be met by others if I let them know what I need."

Steps Six and Seven demand from addicts and coaddicts a complete surrender to their dependency needs. Continuing the spiritual theme of the Twelve Step program, these Steps ask addicts to totally rely on their Higher Power for their recovery. What a challenge for people who lived so many years convinced that they were the only ones who could be trusted to take care of themselves! By asking God and others to meet their needs—thereby giving up control—addicts and coaddicts see a new way to have their needs met. They don't need addiction to deal with anxiety or pain. To be dependent on God and others is an acceptable and preferable way to live.

Addicts and coaddicts fear that they will be let down if they rely on others. With the program they learn that they can be angry when disappointed, which invites further human connection. In the past, they would have responded with an internalized rage, which kept others out and which admitted no need. Even when others occasionally disappoint them, addicts and coaddicts must continue to acknowledge those essential needs, especially to their Higher Power.

Core Belief Four: Sex is my most important need.

Through the Twelve Steps, addicts and coaddicts learn the power the addiction has had in their lives. They discover they do not need the addiction to survive, because what they really wanted could be found in the support of others. They start to live new lives with the focus on healthy human relationships as opposed to sex. They do need the Twelve Step program consistently, however, because of the addiction's power. The conviction that the old obsessions, rituals, and behaviors will bring peace dies hard, especially under stress. Only by living the program daily and experiencing other people's care continuously does that belief diminish.

The Twelve Steps are an ongoing discipline. Steps Ten and Eleven simply make explicit that these Steps are a program that the addict or coaddict lives daily. Step Ten urges them to continue to take personal inventory and when wrong, to promptly admit it. This basic honesty keeps the addict or coaddict rooted in reality and connected in relationships. Step Eleven asks addicts and coaddicts to improve their conscious contact with God through prayer and meditation. The openness to acknowledging human failings, as opposed to concealing them, goes along with a consistent effort to maintain spiritual openness.

In the early days of Alcoholics Anonymous, the Twelfth Step was the one that finally made the program work. Step Twelve requires that addicts carry the message to other addicts as part of their spiritual awakening. They simply pass on what they have received in terms of care and support. Addicts and coaddicts learn that by assisting someone else, all of their learnings are recycled. The Twelfth Step is a measure of how far they have come as well as a reminder of how potent their addiction is.

Addicts and coaddicts find what their obsession could never satisfy: a deep and personal sense of self-worth and value. They can be affirmed and loved, as well as loving and affirming. A rewarding and varied sexual experience within the context of a significant relationship adds nurturing to one's life. Living the program ensures that sexual obsession does not direct one's life. So addicts and coaddicts come to a new belief: "Sex is but one expression of my need and care for others."

Altering the core beliefs is not easy. The Twelve Steps require a rigorous honesty and a commitment to change. For a summary of the key Steps and program principles as they affect the core beliefs, see the chart beginning on page 180, The Twelve Steps and Changing Beliefs.

To borrow from the Big Book of Alcoholics Anonymous, "Some of us have tried to hold on to our old ideas and the result was nil until we let go absolutely." Letting go begins right at the start of the program.

STARTING THE PROGRAM

When Dan's therapist told him that he was sexually addicted, he was outraged! He thought his therapist was exaggerating. Dan was certain his real problem was depression. He was simply down all the time, and he wanted to be happier. True, his life had left a trail of broken relationships and he had some sexual problems, but that was because he was so down all the

time. Yet his therapist had been extremely helpful on a number of issues, so to keep him happy Dan agreed to attend a
couple of meetings of a group that used the Twelve Steps for
sexual compulsivity.

At this first meeting, the group asked that he attend at least
six times. Dan said that he would in order not to make a
scene. Inside, he was convinced that he did not need to be
there. As he listened, he became even more convinced, since
some of the members were struggling with sexual compul-
sions that were alien and even foreign to anything Dan had
ever thought about doing.

Dan set a goal of three meetings—enough to fulfill his therapeutic assignment without prolonging the agony. During his
third meeting, one of the members talked of the notion that
"horniness equals loneliness." Dan listened intently as the
man talked of how he had learned to identify those times
when he was searching for a woman to take care of his anger
and pain. Dan knew exactly the type of panic and desperation
that was being described. For Dan, this was the first realization that maybe the group might fit for him.

Dan attended more meetings. He listened as one man
shared his First Step. He began to realize that his behavior
was really not much different. The exploitation, the efforts to
stop, the painful feelings afterward and the real consequences
fit for him. Soon Dan asked a member of the group to be his
sponsor. His sponsor was an older man who had been in the
program for about four years. Patiently, the sponsor tutored
Dan about how the Steps worked. Dan was amazed at the
complexity and the depth of the Twelve Steps. They were de-
ceptive in their simplicity. Dan recognized that he had much
to learn.

Also, Dan was astounded at how quickly people in the
group became important to him. They listened to him for

many hours on the phone, over coffee, and at lunch. Belonging to the program meant joining up with this network of caring people that extended far beyond the one meeting a week. For the first time in his life, Dan had friends whom he could trust not to abandon him.

Dan found he was sharing parts of himself that he had not even told his therapist, although his group was quick to suggest specific issues that he should bring to therapy. The group stressed that they were not a therapy group, but a Twelve Step program. Most group members recognized, however, that therapy and treatment were important parts of recovery.

STARTING THE FIRST STEP

Dan's sponsor encouraged Dan to start preparing his First Step. Preparation of the First Step involved sharing his sexual history, emphasizing how he was powerless and how his life had become unmanageable. Dan's sponsor told him that he should ask his therapist for assistance as well. "The First Step is too painful to prepare alone," he said. With the help of his sponsor, some group members, and his therapist, Dan started to work. In many ways, it was like preparing for a long journey. Much preparation and planning was necessary before he could start.

Dan's pilgrimage took over three weeks. It was the custom in Dan's group to present a section of the Step each week until it was finished. Some of the sharing was light and humorous. At one point, Dan observed that asking for help was extremely hard. He was the type that would go to an unfamiliar grocery store and, rather than ask where something was, search by himself until he found it. Everyone laughed with Dan about how addicts make life so hard even in the little

OLD CORE BELIEFS	PROGRAM PROVISIONS FOR BOTH ADDICTS AND COADDICTS
1. I am basically a bad, unworthy person.	The program provides the understanding that each member is basically a good person. All learn to separate themselves as individuals from their addiction, which, as a powerful illness, is destroying their lives. When addicts and coaddicts admit the addiction's power, hope emerges from connecting with others and with a Higher Power.
2. No one would love me as I am.	The fellowship of the program surrounds participants with people who have suffered in the same way. They no longer feel unique. They trust and are trusted with personal secrets. They have the opportunity to assess their strengths and weaknesses, as well as to take stock of their own values and behavior. Their new vulnerability allows them the hope of depending on others outside the program. They rediscover the fundamental human processes for restoring relationships through amends and forgiveness.

Figure 7.3

AND CHANGING BELIEFS

KEY STEPS*	NEW BELIEFS	INTEGRATED WORLD
1, 2, 3	I am a worthwhile person deserving of pride.	Addicts and coaddicts have a new sense of pride. Power of the secret world is broken. Identity and integrity return. They no longer need to hide and can become open to each other and to others.
4, 5, 8, 9	I am loved and accepted by people who know me as I am.	Addicts and coaddicts develop a realistic sense of their strengths and weaknesses, of their personal self-worth, and of the limits of their impact on others. They take a new responsibility for their behavior, their behavior becomes more and congruent with their values. They learn that mistakes can be accepted, amends made, and forgiveness received. Addicts and coaddicts can become responsive and responsible members of the human community.

* The numbers correspond to The Twelve Steps of Alcoholics Anonymous Adapted for Sexual Addicts listed on page 170.

OLD CORE BELIEFS	PROGRAM PROVISIONS FOR BOTH ADDICTS AND COADDICTS
3. My needs are never going to be met if I have to depend upon others.	When program members admit their needs, they have their first experience in the care of the fellowship. The program has no conditions or restrictions. Members receive affirmation through admitting their needs. The care they experience provides a basic support, which allows the members to trust a Higher Power and the human community to supply the care they need and to discard the old self-destructive behaviors.
4. Sex is my most important need (addicts), or sex is the most important sign of love (coaddicts).	Addicts and coaddicts learn the power the addiction had in their lives. They discover they do not need the addiction to survive, but they do need the program consistently because of the addiction's power. By recognizing their powerlessness and unmanageablity, addicts and coaddicts start to live new lives that focus on human relationships as opposed to sex. Program members continue to learn about this process through teaching others.

Figure 7.3 *(Continued)*

AND CHANGING BELIEFS (Continued)

KEY STEPS*	NEW BELIEFS	INTEGRATED WORLD
6, 7	My needs can be met by others if I let them know what I need.	By taking more responsibility for themselves, addicts and coaddicts see their roles in having their needs met. Addiction or coaddiction is unnecessary for dealing with anxiety or pain. To be dependent on others is acceptable. When disappointed, appropriate anger invites further human connection, as opposed to rage, which keeps others out.
10, 11, 12	Sex is but one expression of my need and care for others.	Addicts and coaddicts find what their obsession could never discover: a deep and personal sense of self-worth and value. They can be affirmed and loved, as well as loving and affirming. They learn that rewarding and varied sexual experience within the context of significant relationships adds nurturing to one's life. Living the program assures them that sexual obsession does not direct their lives.

* The numbers correspond to The Twelve Steps of Alcoholics Anonymous Adapted for Sexual Addicts listed on page 170.

things. Many parts of Dan's history were very hard to share. Dan found that the most embarrassing example of his compulsivity occurred during his summer job on a farm when he was in college. He had been sexual with farm animals. As he described what he did, his voice became so soft the group strained to listen to him. Then Dan stopped and there was a period of silence. A gentle but strong voice broke the quiet, "Dan, I've done that, too." As he looked up, his eyes full of tears, he looked directly at the other man. There were tears in his eyes, too. Dan was not alone.

The most painful part for Dan to share was about an incident that had occurred two years before Dan had joined the group. Dan had found it exhilarating to sneak into people's houses and watch women undress. He would hide in closets or under beds and then sneak out after everyone was asleep. One of his favorite homes to do this in belonged to some family friends of his parents who had two college-age daughters. One night the mother discovered him hiding in the hall closet. He was profoundly embarrassed because his whole family as well as their friends were involved. In the aftermath, Dan was even more of an outcast in his family.

The group stopped Dan as he was describing all the events that transpired as a result of being discovered. They asked Dan how he felt at the time. He described how he just wanted to die. He acted as if he didn't care, but he was deeply humiliated. Then the group asked him how he felt now. Dan paused. He told them he was angry—angry about being an addict, angry at having to come to the group, angry that he couldn't be just like normal people, angry that he was in such a terrible situation. As the emotions continued, he talked of his sadness about all the people he had hurt, how he had never wanted to be in those situations, and how desperate he had been to stop. He recognized he was powerless, and he felt so alone. His words stopped. All that could be heard now was his deep sobbing, tears that had waited for many years.

Dan learned that night the real depths of his powerlessness, yet he also learned that he was not alone. Life was not a grocery store in which he had to search by himself. Change could occur with the help of a fellowship that cared. Yet, without help and the prerequisite admission that he faced something stronger than he was, he could make no progress.

For months after his First Step, Dan found himself flooded with insight. Other examples and events came to mind—more pieces of a larger puzzle. His group had especially helped him understand the ways he had been abused as a child. His therapist showed Dan how he could translate his new learnings into new behavior. Through his therapy and his program, Dan was achieving a fundamental restructuring of his beliefs as well as an openness to intimacy he had never experienced before.

Even his group noted changes. One member commented to Dan that he could now "see his teeth." He went on to explain that when Dan first came to the group, his smiles were very tight. Now, however, his smiles were relaxed and broad.

Dan was involved soon in his first Twelfth Step call. A Twelfth Step call is when an addict is in need of help and group members meet with the person to assist his or her entry into the program. In this case, the person was sent to the group by the same therapist who had referred Dan. As they met over breakfast, Dan asked the man why he wanted to join the group. He responded by saying that at this point he was not sure that he belonged in the group since he did not know much about it. His therapist, however, was really insistent that he go. Dan remembered his early days and his mind was flooded with realizations about how far he himself had come.

THE IMPACT OF THE FIRST STEP

Dan's experience is typical. People who enter the program go through clear stages. The first is *denial*. Dan did not believe he needed to belong to the program. He thought he could handle his own problems, therefore he kept having them. The second stage is *compliance*. Going through the motions does not indicate acceptance of the program's principles. Rather, people often attend out of duty or even hope that maybe the program might be helpful.

After a time, the new member reaches a third stage, *intellectual acceptance*. The member sees the relevance of the program, empathizes with other members, and makes connections to his or her own behaviors. At this point, the new member starts to develop friendly relationships within the group. Once this support network is established, the member moves to the next stage of *emotional acceptance*. Like Dan, this occurs only after the member has really examined the impact the addiction has had on his or her life.

With that emotional acceptance, the group member experiences an internal surrender to the basic paradox of the First Step. All those years of trying to control the behavior simply intensified the problem. Giving up control, admitting you cannot stop your behavior, acknowledging that this addiction is destroying your life, asking for help—these are the exact opposite actions of what seems natural to do. Yet the Step works.

PREPARATION OF THE STEP

For those of you who are beginning the program, even though you surrender, there is still work to do. Once you have accepted the program's principles, the continuing expansion of awareness leads to a highly creative period for insight into your life. To admit the extremes of your life, and thus become totally exposed, requires a true feeling of support and concern from the group. To be accepted by others is the final rupture of the addictive system. Finally, the First Step will be repeated over and over again in your life, sometimes formally, sometimes in small ways. Each repetition may be done with greater insight, but never with less need. The First Step should be written. You should record as many *specific* examples of powerlessness and unmanageability as possible. Notes should be made of what it was like each time, including feelings, fantasies, concerns, and fears. Do not do this process alone. Share examples with your sponsor, therapist, or group members. Consulting with others builds in accountability, since they can serve as a reality check. Also, these people serve as an important bridge as you sever the bonds of your double life. With their help, you do not have to be stuck in your shame as you write.

Extending your writing can be helpful. Writing in a journal, for example, can add autobiographical depth to your Step. Many treatment programs and therapists require an autobiography of addicts and coaddicts. While the First Step is not designed to deal with your whole life story, there are a number of key life experiences and persons who are very relevant to your addiction. Are there any patterns that emerge? What are the secrets you keep? Who are the significant people who have abandoned you? Recovery starts with identification. By specifying incidents, you can begin to own (to acknowledge and take responsibility for) your addiction. It may help you to reread the early chapters of this book and to review your responses to the various checklists supplied.

For addicts, special attention should be given to the last episode of sexual acting out. Think about exactly what happened, preceded, and followed the incident. What were your feelings and thoughts? If you can establish the date of the incident, that will become your "straight date." In the years to come it will be an important anniversary to mark your progress in the program.

You also need to explore the ways you were victimized as a child or an adolescent. Think of people who were inappropriately sexual with you. Who physically abused you? Who emotionally abused you? Or who neglected you? How did you think and feel at the time? In what ways were you powerless over these events?

Finally, a thorough First Step takes into account the impact of other addictive behaviors like alcoholism, compulsive eating, and workaholism. Avoid causal linkages like "my sexual behavior was the result of my drinking." Rather, note that both addictions were present at the same time. By blaming one addiction on the other, you minimize the addiction's power. By ignoring the presence of other addictions, you dismiss the totality of the addictive process and of your own pain.

Coaddicts use the same process that the addict does, but there are important differences. Obviously, coaddicts are preoccupied and obsessed with the addicts' behavior. Coaddicts have to admit powerlessness over the addicts. Coaddicts will feel angry about being connected to an addict. Abuse issues and other addictions are important factors for the coaddicts as well.

Many addicts and coaddicts find that professional assistance accelerates recovery. Treatment programs and therapists offer a number of advantages. First, if they are skilled in addiction and knowledgeable in the Twelve Step program, they can help you focus on the fundamental changes necessary to stop your illness. Second, professionals can assist families in restructuring their relationships with skills and perspectives additional to what the Twelve Steps offer. Finally, they can attend to the mental health issues that are often concurrent with the addiction.

THE SAFE FORMULA

Unlike an alcoholic who can abstain and maintain sobriety, the sexual addict has to face the fact of his or her own sexuality. Like the overeater, recovery does not mean the elimination of fundamental human processes. Celibacy does not resolve the problem. The question emerges for addicts as to how they determine when their sexual behavior is addictive.

The following formula is suggested as a guideline. Signs of compulsive sexuality are when the behavior can be described as follows:

1. It is a *secret*. Anything that cannot pass public scrutiny will create the shame of a double life.
2. It is *abusive* to self or others. Anything that is exploitive or harmful to others or degrades oneself will activate the addictive system.
3. It is used to avoid or is a source of painful *feelings*. If sexuality is used to alter moods or results in painful mood shifts, it is clearly part of the addictive process.
4. It is *empty* of a caring, committed relationship. Fundamental to the whole concept of addiction and recovery is the healthy dimension of human relationships. The addict runs a great risk by being sexual outside of a committed relationship.

The advantage of the SAFE (Secret, Abusive, Feelings, Empty) formula is that it is built on the basic concept of addiction and is in the spirit of the Twelve Steps. It requires a ruthless honesty, given that the addict's sanity is at stake. Using the group or a sponsor as an ongoing reality check can help keep the addict "safe." You may wish to use The Addict's Worksheet on pages 192 and 193 as a means for thinking about your own behavior.

JOINING A GROUP

Seeking a Twelve Step group feels difficult, because by searching you admit you have a problem. Start by checking local community referral agencies or phone services. Private therapists, pastors, social service agencies, and Alcoholics Anonymous and Al-Anon (for family members of alcoholics) programs are also good resources. You may even be fortunate enough to have a treatment program in your area. Many local alcoholism programs are now offering help for sexual addicts. You could then join a Twelve Step group after you have finished treatment.

Some cities as well as rural areas have a large number of groups, including groups for family members and women addicts. If that is true in your area, remember that each group has its own unique character. Some have a style or composition that may not be a good match for you, so continue searching. However, remember the six-meeting rule, because the problem may not be with the group but with your denial.

If you become discouraged, find a copy of the Big Book of Alcoholics Anonymous. Read the first eleven chapters, which tell of the early days of AA in the late 1930s, when AA had fewer than a hundred members. Look specifically at chapter 5, "How It Works," which says in part:

> Rarely have we seen a person fail who has thoroughly followed our path. Those who do not recover are people

who cannot or will not completely give themselves to this simple program, usually men and women who are constitutionally incapable of being honest with themselves. . . . Many of us exclaimed, "What an order! I can't go through with it." Do not be discouraged. No one among us has been able to maintain anything like perfect adherence to these principles. We are not saints. The point is that we are willing to grow along spiritual lines.

The following exercise will assist you in thinking about your addiction. You may wish to use a separate sheet or journal to complete the tasks required. The first task is to make two lists. One list should record sexual experiences in your life that have been degrading or exploitive. The other list should contain experiences that have been enriching or life-enhancing. Take care to be absolutely honest with yourself. Also make your descriptions as specific as possible.

DEGRADING OR EXPLOITIVE BEHAVIOR

1. _____

_____

2. _____

_____

3. _____

_____

4. _____

_____

5. _____

_____

6. _____

_____

7. _____

_____

8. _____

_____

Figure 7.4

WORKSHEET

Now note the common feelings, attitudes, and situations in each list. For example, did the activities in the first list involve secrecy or dishonesty? How are they different? What guidelines do the lists indicate in terms of addictive behavior that you need to stop? Share these with someone who understands your program (e.g., a sponsor, therapist, or group member).

ENRICHING OR LIFE-ENHANCING BEHAVIOR

1. _____

_____

_____

2. _____

_____

_____

3. _____

_____

_____

4. _____

_____

_____

5. _____

_____

_____

6. _____

_____

_____

7. _____

_____

_____

8. _____

_____

_____

CHAPTER 8

The Future Is Conditional

◻ ◻ ◻

I am larger, better than I thought.
I did not know I held so much goodness.

—Walt Whitman

John was a town councilman. He had been an effective and well-liked leader. John was also a sexual addict, but had received treatment and had been in a Twelve Step program for two years. A newspaper reporter had dug up an old police report that had accused John of exposing himself. The reporter described the accusation in an article that quickly brought demands for John's resignation. When John resigned, an outstanding community member appointed by the council replaced him. The irony was that John's replacement was from his own Twelve Step group.

A second story relates the experience of the schoolteacher who was sexual with students. When the facts became known, the community stood behind the teacher. He had made an enormous contribution to the welfare of the town. Townspeople sensitively stood behind the teacher, helped him get treatment, and kept his job open.

The contrast in public attitudes is obvious. Unfortunately, most people react as the townspeople did in John's case. Part of the problem is that for the public to understand the sexual addiction, the majority would have to conduct painful self-appraisals of their own beliefs and family rules. Because of the many social factors, professionals can only guess at the extent of sexual compulsivity. Addicts simply do not volunteer that information. Nor is there public pride in recovery. A sex addict cannot, in our day and time, proudly announce his or her recovery, as alcoholics now can.

Sexual addicts need to remember the decades of struggle that alcoholics had to go through in order to earn public acceptance of their illness. Even now, large parts of the population still see alcoholism as a matter of moral degeneracy. We are perhaps decades away from a public understanding of the problem of sexual addiction. The surest way to gain public support will be to document the cost—the cost to addicts, their families, the community, business, and industry.

A military chaplain describes a situation that illustrates the cost. On an overseas base, one man's sexual binges had a serious impact on his work. He contracted a particularly vicious form of venereal disease seventeen times during a two-year tour. When the situation was brought to the attention of the base commander, his initial response was that he could not act on something that was so clearly a personal matter. The chaplain pointed out that the venereal disease was so severe each time that the man had lost on the average four days of work per treatment. The base commander understood the chaplain's point. Together they worked with the man to get him to the help he needed.

The sexual addiction affects job productivity and performance. Distraction, time loss, unmanageability, poor decision making—all are commonly reported by addicts. Each addict's story, however, makes a unique statement about the cost:

- the manager of a large retail outlet who was fired when

> he completed a two-month term in jail for incest

- the woman who left her husband and children to meet her online cybersex partner, only to discover the partner was actually a fifteen-year-old boy
- the bank executive who discovered during treatment that his job promotion had been held back for years because of his sexual addiction
- the laid-off truck driver who sold food stamps on the black market to buy gas in order to cruise eight to sixteen hours each day looking for women
- the cab driver with seven children who could not renew his license because of an arrest for sexual misconduct
- the child advocate who had to confess child abuse
- the beauty shop owner who lost his business because of involvement with clients
- the owner of a family appliance business who lost his wife and his business because of incest
- the forty-five-year-old painter who spent a total of twenty-five years in prison for various sex-related charges
- the nursing home attendant who requested not to work with female patients because of his fears of obsession

Employers have a special perspective on the costs of sexual addiction. They can see the patterns. For example, the bishop who has to move yet another young clergyman with a habit of being sexual with parishioners to a different parish, the superintendent who hears still another story about the seventh-grade math teacher who masturbates in the classroom, and the executive whose firm faces a sexual harassment suit against one of his employees because of sexual behavior. All these examples have in common the perspective of an emerging pattern of sexual addiction. Employers can also put pressure on the addict to seek help.

Procedures that are now routine for intervening with alcoholics in most professional, business, and industrial settings can be utilized for the sexual addict as well. Already many employee assistance programs are recognizing that there are valuable, talented people who cannot help themselves because of their illness. In fact, many alcoholism programs are developing special tracks for sexual compulsiveness to respond to industry's need. This is especially appropriate given that many suffer from both sexual addiction and addiction to alcohol or other drugs.

The addict can be helped in many ways, including

- public awareness of the sexual addiction as a tragic illness that can be stopped in most cases
- elimination of jokes that degrade people's struggle with their sexual compulsivity, such as "flasher" jokes, dirty-bookstore jokes
- support by local community agencies, including churches, schools, and hospitals to allow meetings in their facilities
- honest appraisal of the problem by judges so that treatment is one of the consequences
- prevention programs that promote family health and communication, especially about sexual issues
- treatment providers who extend services not only to the addicts but also to family members
- clinicians who are not bound by narrow categories that blind them to the overall picture, including the interconnectedness, of compulsive behavior
- lawyers, ministers, and physicians who can see the signs of the addiction and can intervene in the destructive cycle

- police who neither dismiss nor overreact to the addict's problem
- alcohol addiction counselors who are willing to apply their special skills to multiple addictions
- child protection workers who recognize that all members of the family are desperate
- researchers who, using critical scientific standards, take on the difficult task of expanding understanding

By making these efforts to help sexual addicts and coaddicts, we can support the spirit of the Twelve Step program. If this book contributes toward that end, it will have accomplished its purpose: to create legitimacy for those courageous people who wish to face their sexual compulsivity for what it truly is—an addiction. With our help, those addicts will be truly able to say, in the words of Walt Whitman:

I am larger, better than I thought.
I did not know I held so much goodness.

Notes

Preface to the 2001 Edition

1. P. Carnes, "The Presidential Diagnosis," editorial, *Sexual Addiction and Compulsivity: The Journal of Treatment and Prevention* 5, no. 3 (1998); M. Isikoff, *Uncovering Clinton: A Reporter's Story* (New York: Crown Publishers, 1999).

2. A. Cooper, D. Delmonico, and R. Burg, "Cybersex Users, Abusers, and Compulsives: New Findings and Implications," *Sexual Addiction and Compulsivity: The Journal of Treatment and Prevention* 7, nos. 1–2 (2000).

Chapter 1: The Addiction Cycle

1. M. MacAuliffe and R. MacAuliffe, *The Essentials of Chemical Dependency* (Minneapolis, Minn.: American Chemical Dependency Society, 1975).

2. P. Carnes, *Don't Call It Love: Recovery from Sexual Addiction* (New York: Bantam Books, 1992).

3. For a description of the literature describing the interaction of drugs, alcohol, and sexual compulsivity, see P. Carnes, *Contrary to Love: Helping the Sexual Addict* (Center City, Minn.: Hazelden, 1989), the companion volume to this book.

4. Carnes, *Don't Call It Love.*

5. A. Washton, "Cocaine May Trigger Sexual Compulsivity," *U.S. Journal of Drug and Alcohol Dependency* 13, no. 6 (1989): 8.

6. The concept of concurrent addictions is being more widely accepted. William R. Miller, for example, writes: "What do the following have in common: alcoholism, obesity, smoking, drug abuse, and compulsive gambling? Until a few years ago, these were thought of as relatively independent and separate problem areas. Psychologists, psychiatrists,

social workers, and other mental health professionals have often specialized in the treatment of one of these behaviors, but few have extended their therapy and research efforts to cover more than one or two of these disorders. In addition, specialists in each of these areas have worked in relative isolation from one another, seldom communicating with each other about treatment and research issues. The past few years, however, have witnessed a remarkable amount of growth and change in professional knowledge within these areas. The emergent concept of 'the addictive behaviors' points to possible commonalities among these seemingly diverse problems." Miller, *The Addictive Behaviors* (New York: Pergamon Press, 1980), 3. For the professional, a useful journal committed to this subject is *Addictive Diseases: An International Journal* (Spectrum Publications, 192nd St., Flushing, N.Y.).

7. Carnes, *Don't Call It Love*; P. Carnes and K. Adams, *The Clinical Management of Sex Addiction* (Philadelphia: Taylor and Francis, 2001).

8. For an excellent summary of this literature, see Warren Shaffer and Alan Anderson, "Group Approaches to Counseling," chapter 8 of *Handbook of Counseling Psychology*, ed. Steven D. Brown and Robert W. Lent (New York: John Wiley, 2001).

Chapter 2: The Levels of Addiction

1. For readers who wish to read further on sexual behavior during phases of transition, see Gail Sheehy, *Passages: Predictable Crises in Adult Life* (New York: Dutton, 1974); Robert S. Weiss, *Marital Separation* (New York: Basic Books, 1975); David M. Reed, "Sexual Behavior in the Separated, Divorced, and Widowed," in *The Sexual Experience*, ed. Benjamin J. Sadock, Harold I. Kaplan, and Alfred M. Freedman (Baltimore, Md.: Williams and Wilkins, 1976); Peter

Blos, *The Adolescent Passage* (New York: International Universities Press, 1979).

2. An example of the prevailing belief is a statement from Lt. Jim Bullard's *Looking Forward to Being Attacked* (Memphis Police Department): "Exhibitionists generally are introverted and shy. They are bashful. They are almost never dangerous."

3. From an unpublished manuscript presented at the First Annual Conference for the Treatment of Sexual Aggressives, July 1977.

4. Neil Malamuth, "Rapists and Normal Men," *Treatment for Sexual Aggressives News* 5 (1982): 1.

5. Donald E. MacNamara and Edward Sagarin, *Sex, Crime, and the Law* (New York: Free Press, 1978).

6. For a review of literature on this subject, see Carnes, *Contrary to Love.*

Chapter 3: Cybersex and Addictive Behavior

1. Cooper, Delmonico, and Burg, "Cybersex Users, Abusers, and Compulsives: New Findings and Implications," *Sexual Addiction and Compulsivity: The Journal of Treatment and Prevention* 7, nos. 1–2 (2000): 5–30. This whole issue of the journal was dedicated to cybersex addiction.

2. H. Fisher, "Lust, Attraction, Attachment: Biology and Evolution of the Three Primary Emotion Systems for Mating, Reproduction, and Parenting," *Journal of Sex Education and Therapy* 25, no. 1 (2000): 96–104.

3. J. Money, *Lovemaps: Clinical Concepts of Sexual/Erotic Health and Pathology* (Amherst, N.Y.: Prometheus Books, 1989).

Chapter 4: The Family and the Addict's World

1. Nick Coleman, "Brothers Sentenced in Sex Case," *Minneapolis Tribune*, January 20, 1982.

2. H. Eist and A. Mandel, "Family Treatment of On-going Incest Behavior," *Family Process* 7 (1968): 216.

3. Julia Sherman, "The Coatlicue Complex: A Source of Irrational Reactions against Women," *Transactional Analysis Journal* 5 (1975): 2.

Chapter 6: The Belief System

1. Helen Block Lewis, *Psychic War in Men and Women* (New York: New York University Press, 1976), vii.

2. Warren Farrell, "We Teach Men to Be Rapists," *Sexuality Today* 1, no. 32 (1978): 3.

3. Rollo May, *Power and Innocence: A Search for the Sources of Innocence* (New York: Norton, 1972).

4. Richard Bandler and John Grinder, *The Structure of Magic*, vols. 1 and 2 (Palo Alto, Calif.: Science and Behavior Books, 1975).

Chapter 7: Twelve Steps to Recovery

1. Sandra Boodman, "Former Educator Sentenced to Jail," *Washington Post*, April 28, 1982.

2. Ernest Becker, *The Denial of Death* (New York: Free Press, 1973).

Resource Guide

For the latest information on what is available for sex addicts, go to www.sexhelp.com. This Web site includes archived articles, annotated book lists, a schedule of important events, and links to other key Web sites. Additional important Web sites include www.gentlepath.com for publications, www.addictionresearch.com for current research, and www.recoveryzone.com for recovery resources. For general information on sex addiction, contact the Society for the Advancement of Sexual Health, P.O. Box 725544, Atlanta, GA 31139, 770-541-9912, or access their Web site at www.sash.net. In addition, individual fellowships publish literature and periodicals. A list is provided at the conclusion of this guide.

For information on certified sex addiction therapists in your local area, go to www.sexhelp.com or call 1-800-708-1796. For information on workshops, conferences, and retreats with Dr. Carnes, please call 1-800-708-1796 or write to Gentle Path, P.O. Box 3172, Carefree, AZ 85377. For information on audiotapes, videotapes, and other publications authored by Dr. Carnes, call 1-800-708-1796 or write to Gentle Path Press, P.O. Box 3172, Carefree, AZ 85377.

Hope and Recovery: A Twelve Step Guide for Healing from Compulsive Sexual Behavior (Hazelden, 1987) has long been a useful guide. For those beginning recovery, *Facing the Shadow: Starting Sexual and Relationship Recovery* (Gentle Path Press, 2005) is designed as an accompanying workbook for *Out of the Shadows*. Also, Dr. Carnes, along with David Delmonico and Elizabeth Griffin, has written *In the Shadows of the Net: Breaking Free of Compulsive Online Sexual Behavior* (Hazelden, 2001). Other books by Dr. Carnes include *Don't Call It Love: Recovery from Sexual Addiction* (Bantam, 1992), *Contrary to*

Love: Helping the Sexual Addict (Hazelden, 1989), *A Gentle Path through the Twelve Steps: The Classic Guide for All People in the Process of Recovery* (Hazelden, 1993), *Sexual Anorexia: Overcoming Sexual Self-Hatred* (Hazelden, 1997), *The Betrayal Bond: Breaking Free of Exploitive Relationships* (Health Communications, 1997), and *Open Hearts: Renewing Relationships with Recovery, Romance, and Reality* (Gentle Path Press, 1999).

Other helpful books by other authors include *Answers in the Heart: Daily Meditations for Men and Women Recovering from Sex Addiction* (Hazelden, 1989). Other contributions are Anne Wilson Schaef's highly readable *Escape from Intimacy: Untangling the "Love" Addictions* (Harper San Francisco, 1990) and Ralph Earle's powerful *Lonely All the Time: Recognizing, Understanding, and Overcoming Sex Addiction* (Pocket Books, 1998). Add Charlotte Kasl's important book *Women, Sex, and Addiction: A Search for Love and Power* (HarperCollins, 1990) and Jed Diamond's *Looking for Love in All the Wrong Places: Overcoming Romantic and Sexual Addictions* (Avon, 1989), and we find a complete bookshelf being created for recovering sex addicts.

For survivors of sexual abuse, many resources have appeared. Mic Hunter's *Abused Boys: The Neglected Victims of Sexual Abuse* (Fawcett Books, 1991) is a groundbreaking effort to create resources for men who were abused. Wendy Maltz, whose *Incest and Sexuality: A Guide to Understanding and Healing* (Lexington Books, 1987) is already regarded as a classic, is also the author of *The Sexual Healing Journey: A Guide for Survivors of Sexual Abuse* (Quill, 2001). This superb book provides concrete ways for a victim to reintegrate the sexual self. Similarly, Ellen Bass and Laura Davis have created classics in their *Courage to Heal: A Guide for Women Survivors of Child Sexual Abuse* (HarperPerennial, 1994), both book and workbook. Their book *Allies in Healing: When the Person You Love Was Sexually Abused as a Child* (HarperPerennial, 1991) is extremely well crafted and fills an important gap as a resource for the spouse of a survivor. Probably one of the most important books in this category is Dr. Patricia Love's *Emotional Incest Syndrome: What to Do When a Parent's Love Rules Your Life* (Bantam, 1991). This book has been an eye-opener for many. For sex addicts who have emotional incest issues, Kenneth M. Adams's *Silently Seduced: When Parents Make Their Children Partners* (Health Communications, 1991) has been a gift.

For adult children of alcoholics and other addictions, the sexual issues are legion. A fine guide to integrating recovery and sexuality is *Aching for Love: The Sexual Drama of the Adult Child* by Mary A. Klausner and Bobbie Hasselbring (Harper San Francisco, 1990). Claudia Black's *Double Duty* (MAC Publishing, 1990) is very helpful about sexual issues, as well as others. For women, Stephanie Covington has written an excellent guide called *Awakening Your Sexuality: A Guide for Recovering Women* (Hazelden, 2000).

For family members of sex addicts, Jennifer Schneider has updated her wonderful book *Back from Betrayal: Recovering from His Affairs* (Recovery Resources Press, 2001).

On intimacy issues as they affect sexual behavior, two highly regarded and useful books are Harriet Goldhor Lerner's *The Dance of Intimacy: A Woman's Guide to Courageous Acts of Change in Key Relationships* (HarperCollins, 1990) and *The Dance of Anger: A Woman's Guide to Changing the Patterns of Intimate Relationships* (HarperCollins, 1997). I also like John H. Driggs and Stephen E. Finn's *Intimacy between Men: How to Find and Keep Gay Love Relationships* (Plume, 1991) for its discussion of homosexuality and intimacy.

A task for many clients is resolving issues in the family,

especially sexual ones. *Dear Dad: Letters from an Adult Child* (Penguin, 1991) by Louie Anderson is a good model for the courage it takes. John Bradshaw's *Homecoming: Reclaiming and Championing Your Inner Child* (Bantam, 1992) is filled with strategies for resolution of family of origin issues and is a testimony to the possibilities of the human spirit. Melody Beattie's *The Language of Letting Go* (Hazelden, 1990) is a gentle way to personal resolution. For journaling strategies, no better book exists than Christina Baldwin's *Life's Companion: Journal Writing as a Spiritual Quest* (Bantam, 1998).

Facing Shame: Families in Recovery (Norton, 1989) by Merle Fossum and Marilyn Mason was intended for therapists and is one of the best books available on family therapy and addictions. It is highly readable, however, and most readers will find it filled with extraordinary insight on family functioning.

A final suggestion: in many ways therapy and recovery are like reparenting, wherein we are adding new voices to supplant the old destructive ones. Good books can add new messages and empower you to be able to affirm your sexuality from within. Sharing reading with your partner and in your groups can only add to your understanding and intimacy. The gift of recovery means we no longer have to do things in isolation.

To arrange for seminars, conferences, workshops, or lectures by Patrick Carnes, call 1-800-708-1796.

NATIONAL ADDRESSES OF TWELVE STEP
PROGRAMS FOR SEX ADDICTION

For the addict:
The following programs differ primarily in their definition of "sexual sobriety." In cities when more than one of these programs has meetings, many addicts attend them interchangeably.

Sexaholics Anonymous (SA)
P.O. Box 3565
Brentwood, TN 37024
615-331-6062 or Toll-free: 866-424-8777
E-mail: saico@sa.org

Sex and Love Addicts Anonymous (SLAA)
P.O. Box 338
Norwood, MA 02062
781-255-8825
E-mail: slaafws@aol.com
Web: www.slaafws.org

Sex Addicts Anonymous (SAA)
P.O. Box 70949
Houston, TX 77270
713-869-4902 or (within U.S.A. and Canada) 800-477-8191
E-mail: info@saa-recovery.org
Web: www.sexaa.org

Sexual Compulsives Anonymous (SCA)
Old Chelsea Station
P.O. Box 1585
New York, NY 10011
800-977-HEAL
Web: www.sca-recovery.org/index.html

For the partner or family member:
The following two programs, both for families and friends of sex addicts, have no significant differences in their philosophy. Generally, only one or the other is well represented in any one city.

S-Anon International Family Groups
P.O. Box 17294
Nashville, TN 37217
615-833-3152 or Toll-free: 800-210-8141
E-mail: saifg@sanon.org
Web: sanon@sanon.org

Codependents of Sex Addicts (COSA)
P.O. Box 14537
Minneapolis, MN 55414
763-537-6904
E-mail: cosa@shore.net
Web: www2.primushost.com/~cosa

For couples:
Recovering Couples Anonymous (RCA)
P.O. Box 11029
Oakland, CA 94611
781-794-1456 or Toll-free: 1-877-663-2317
E-mail: info@Recovering-Couples.org
Web: www.recovering-couples.org

For information on education, conferences, and referrals:
The Society for the Advancement of Sexual Health
P.O. Box 725544
Atlanta, GA 31139
770-541-9912
Web: www.sash.net

For peer-reviewed medical literature about sex addiction
and compulsivity:
*Sexual Addiction and Compulsivity: The Journal of Treatment and
Prevention*
215-625-8900
E-mail: ppagano@taylorandfrancis.com

For more resources on sex addiction:
www.sexhelp.com

For complete database and bibliography of information on
sexual addiction:
www.addictionresearch.com

RECOMMENDED READING LIST

Carnes, P. J. *Don't Call It Love: Recovery from Sexual Addiction.*
New York: Bantam Books, 1992.
———. "Addiction or Compulsion: Politics or Illness?" *Sexual
Addiction and Compulsivity: The Journal of Treatment and
Prevention* 3, no. 2 (1996).
Earle, R., M. Earle, and K. Osborn, *Sexual Addiction Case
Studies and Management.* N.p.:Brunner/Mazel, 1995.
Goodman, A. *Sexual Addiction: An Integrated Approach.*
Madison, Conn.: International Universities Press, 1998.
Schneider, J. P. *Back from Betrayal.* N.p.:Recovery Resources
Press, 2001.

Index

About the Author

Patrick J. Carnes, Ph.D., C.A.S., is the former clinical director for sexual disorders services at The Meadows in Wickenburg, Arizona. Dr. Carnes is a nationally known speaker on addiction and recovery issues, as well as the sole author or contributing author of the following books on addiction: *Understanding Us* (1980); *Out of the Shadows: Understanding Sexual Addiction* (2001); *Contrary to Love: Helping the Sexual Addict* (1989); *A Gentle Path through the Twelve Steps: The Classic Guide for All People in the Process of Recovery* (1993); *Don't Call It Love: Recovery from Sexual Addiction* (1992); *Sexual Anorexia: Overcoming Sexual Self-Hatred* (1997); *The Betrayal Bond: Breaking Free of Exploitive Relationships* (1997); *Open Hearts: Renewing Relationships with Recovery, Romance, and Reality* (1999); *In the Shadows of the Net: Breaking Free of Compulsive Online Sexual Behavior* (2001); *Facing the Shadow: Starting Sexual and Relationship Recovery* (2001); and *The Recovery Zone* (2001).

Additionally, Dr. Carnes serves on the National Advisory Board of the American Academy of Health Care Providers in the Addictive Disorders, a national certification organization for clinical professionals. Dr. Carnes is the focus of a twelve-part PBS series on addictions called *Contrary to Love*.

Previously, Dr. Carnes designed and created the country's first inpatient sexual dependency facility at Golden Valley Health Center in Minneapolis. He was a founding board member of the National Council on Sexual Addiction and Compulsivity (NCSAC), a community and professional organization for public awareness about sexual health.

Carnes received his doctorate in education and counseling from the University of Minnesota.

About Hazelden Publishing

As part of the Hazelden Betty Ford Foundation, Hazelden Publishing offers both cutting-edge educational resources and inspirational books. Our print and digital works help guide individuals in treatment and recovery, and their loved ones. Professionals who work to prevent and treat addiction also turn to Hazelden Publishing for evidence-based curricula, digital content solutions, and videos for use in schools, treatment programs, correctional programs, and electronic health records systems. We also offer training for implementation of our curricula.

Through published and digital works, Hazelden Publishing extends the reach of healing and hope to individuals, families, and communities affected by addiction and related issues.

For more information about Hazelden publications,
please call **800-328-9000**
or visit us online at **hazelden.org/bookstore.**